Rheumatism for Nurses and Remedial Therapists

Rheumatism for Nurses and Remedial Therapists

V. WRIGHT MD FRCP
Professor of Rheumatology, Rheumatism Research Unit, School of Medicine, University of Leeds.

and

IAN HASLOCK MD
Consultant Rheumatologist, South Tees Health District.

with the collaboration of
B. CHAMPNEY SRN RNT
Principal Nursing Officer (Education), General Infirmary, Leeds.

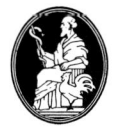

WILLIAM HEINEMANN MEDICAL BOOKS LTD
London

First published 1977

© V. Wright, I. Haslock and B. Champney 1977

ISBN 0 433 37020 3

Printed in Great Britain at
The Lavenham Press Limited, Lavenham, Suffolk.

Acknowledgements

We are grateful for permission to reproduce certain diagrams from the *Handbooks for Patients* produced by the Arthritis and Rheumatism Association and from their slide collection, and from 'Care of the Feet' and 'Avoiding Back Trouble' published by the Consumers' Association. Dr A. St. J. Dixon kindly allowed us to use certain diagrams from *Arthritis and Physical Medicine* published by Licht. The figure on pathology of osteoarthrosis is reproduced by permission from the Clinical Slide Collection on the Rheumatic Diseases produced by the Arthritis Foundation, New York, 1972.

We are grateful for helpful discussion on the Physiotherapy chapter to Mrs J. Hawkes, Miss M. Jackson and Mr R. Webster; and on the Occupational Therapy chapter to Miss S. Calvert, Miss J. Fogden and Miss G. Thornley. We are also deeply indebted to many nursing colleagues in this field, particularly our Ward Sisters, Miss E. J. Boyington, Miss K. M. Bradley, Mrs M. Cook, Miss R. Cox, Miss F. M. Ellis, Miss M. I. S. Hutchinson, Mrs M. Mulloy and Mrs B. Yung.

Contents

1.	Structure and Function of Joints	1
2.	Rheumatic Diseases in the Community	12
3.	Rheumatoid Arthritis	21
4.	Osteoarthrosis	36
5.	Infective Arthritis	47
6.	Ankylosing Spondylitis	56
7.	Degenerative Disease of the Spine	65
8.	Non-articular Rheumatism	82
9.	Shoulder Disorders	89
10.	The Diffuse Connective Tissue Diseases	96
11.	Rheumatic Fever	107
12.	Gout	115
13.	Disorders of the Foot	126
14.	Miscellaneous Types of Arthritis	135
15.	Physiotherapy	144
16.	Occupational Therapy	153
17.	Rehabilitation	167
18.	Prevention	176
19.	Laboratory Investigations	183
20.	Nursing Care	194
21.	Drug Therapy in Rheumatic Diseases	204
22.	Surgery	223
	Index	235

Preface

The rheumatic diseases are among the commonest of all diseases, costing the nation millions of pounds from the economic point of view and exerting a tremendous toll of suffering in the community. Many of these sufferers are admitted to hospital for treatment or attend the outpatient clinic, physiotherapy and occupational therapy departments. Still more require further help at home.

Moreover, rheumatic patients may be stricken with some other illness. For instance, a patient with ankylosing spondylitis may require an extensive excision of bowel for unrelated cancer. The associated arthritis may easily be overlooked with disastrous results. The total person must always be treated.

The importance of the subject is recognised in the teaching given to student and pupil nurses, and students in the remedial professions. The Joint Board of Clinical Nursing Studies has published details of a post-basic nursing course in the subject. It is for these students that this book is primarily written. However, a medical student who knew its contents would be unlikely to fail his final examination due to deficient knowledge in rheumatology (at least in Leeds!). Social workers dealing with the physically handicapped could study it with profit to themselves and their clients.

1
Structure and Function of Joints

Introduction
Types of Synovial Joints
General Structure
  The Cartilage
  Synovial membrane
  Synovial fluid
  Capsule
  Nerve supply
  Blood supply
  Muscles
  Intra-articular structures
  Ligaments
  Connective tissue
Loads
Lubrication

Introduction

Man has over 300 joints in his body. Through the centuries they have been classified in two main groups:
  1. synostosis
  2. synovial (diarthrodial).

Where two bones are united by fibrous tissue or cartilage this is called a synostosis. Some authors would, in fact, recognise fibrous joints and cartilaginous joints as quite separate. Examples of synostoses are found between the bones of the skull, and in infancy movement between these can be readily detected. Another example is the symphysis pubis, where the two halves of the pelvis meet anteriorly. During pregnancy, due to the circulation of relaxin, this fibrous tissue may soften to allow expansion of the pelvis during delivery. At times this may cause undue separation and the mother experiences much pain on walking during the last three months of pregnancy. Another example is the costochondral junction between the rib and the cartilage which unites the rib to the sternum in the front. There are diseases in which these junctions may become painful.

The commonest type of joint in the body, however, is the synovial (diarthrodial) joint between the two bones. This is shown diagrammatically in Fig. 1.1. Synovial joints consist essentially of bone ends capped by cartilage, contained within a fibrous capsule: this is lined by synovium, which secretes lubricant fluid (synovial fluid). There are over 260 of these joints in the body and we shall be mainly concerned with

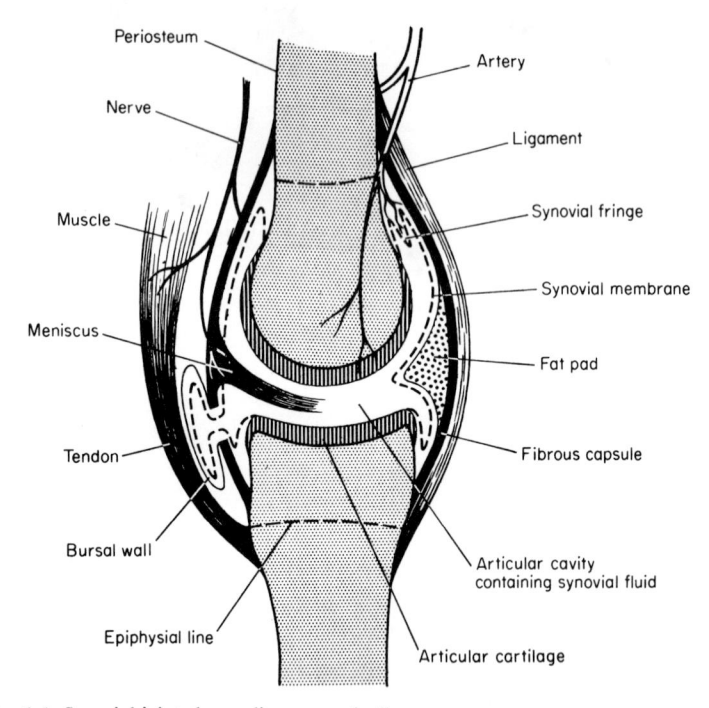

Fig. 1.1. Synovial joint shown diagrammatically.

them in this chapter, since these are the joints usually involved in rheumatic disorders. These joints are remarkable bearings, far better than any engineer has produced, with a sliding ability better than glass rubbing on ice. Their main function is to allow the movement of one segment of the body on another in a creature supported by an internal skeleton. The ability of weightbearing joints to function without trouble for the lifespan of most users is remarkable when the size of the forces encountered is considered; these may be many times bodyweight in certain activities, and at times may be borne by an area as small as a postage stamp.

Types of Synovial Joints

In structural terms the joints are:
- plain—e.g. inter-metacarpal (Fig. 1.2a);
- ball and socket (spheroidal)—e.g. hip (Fig. 1.2b);
- ellipsoid—e.g. metacarpo-phalangeal (Fig. 1.2c);
- hinge—e.g. humero-ulnar (Fig. 1.2d);
- condylar—e.g. knee (Fig. 1.2e);
- pivot (trochoid)—e.g. superior radio-ulnar (Fig. 1.2f);
- saddle or sellar—e.g. 1st carpo-metacarpal (Fig. 1.2g);

As well as allowing movement the joint must maintain stability. The structure of the hip is a good example of the means of support of a joint. It is kept together partly by the close fit of the spherical femoral head within the hip socket (acetabulum), which is extended around its margin by fibrocartilage (labra). Strong ligaments, such as the iliofemoral, and short muscles, such as the glutei medius and minimus, acting externally provide further strength. Finally, the fibrous outer envelope of the joint assists in keeping the entire structure intact. If the structures within the joint are destroyed, it becomes unstable. This is commonly seen in the knee where arthritis destroying the shape of the joint may enable it to be wobbled from side to side. This gives the impression that the ligaments of the joint have become slack but this is not so because, if the joint structure is restored by the insertion of artificial material to make a new joint, stability is regained without anything being done to the ligaments.

General Structure

The cartilage

The cartilage which caps the bone is white and glistening, as may be seen by looking at bones in the butcher's shop. Cartilage is a sponge-like material with many minute pores, which allow synovial fluid to be pumped in and out; in this way the cartilage is nourished, since it has no blood supply. This tissue is not very firm and could be compared with the firmness of the rubber of a car tyre, whereas bone has a firmness like wood.

Synovial membrane

Surrounding the joint completely is synovial membrane; this is a vascular structure, which readily becomes inflamed by any irritation, whether it be an infection or some other local irritant. It secretes synovial fluid into the joint cavity. In certain conditions when the lining becomes inflamed, a surgeon may remove it (synovectomy), but he is never able to excise it completely and the tissue quickly regrows.

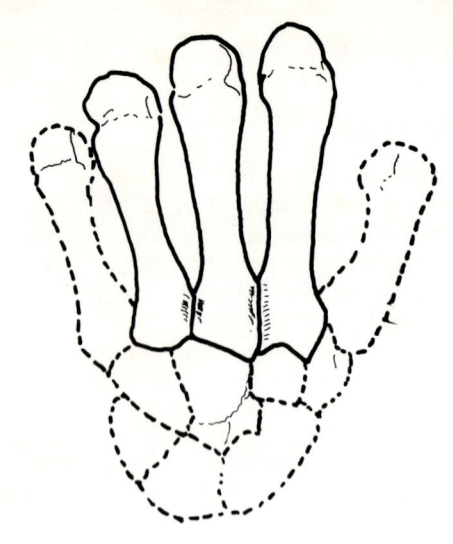

Fig. 1.2a. Plain joint—inter-metacarpal joint.

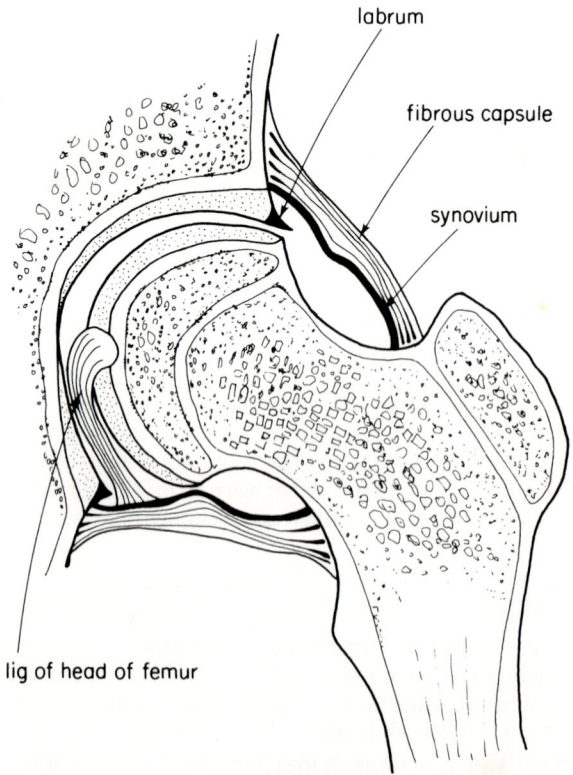

Fig. 1.2b. Ball and socket (spheroidal) joint—hip.

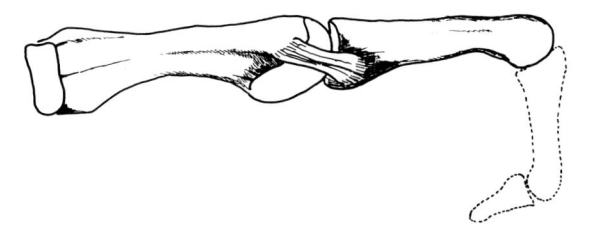

Fig. 1.2c. Ellipsoid joint—metacarpo-phalangeal joint.

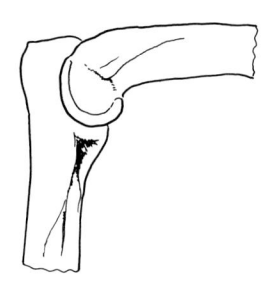

Fig. 1.2d. Hinge joint—humero-ulnar joint.

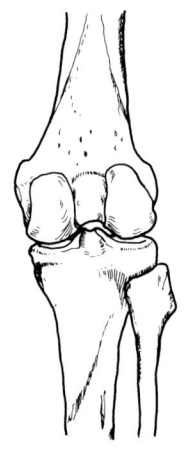

Fig. 1.2e. Condylar joint—knee.

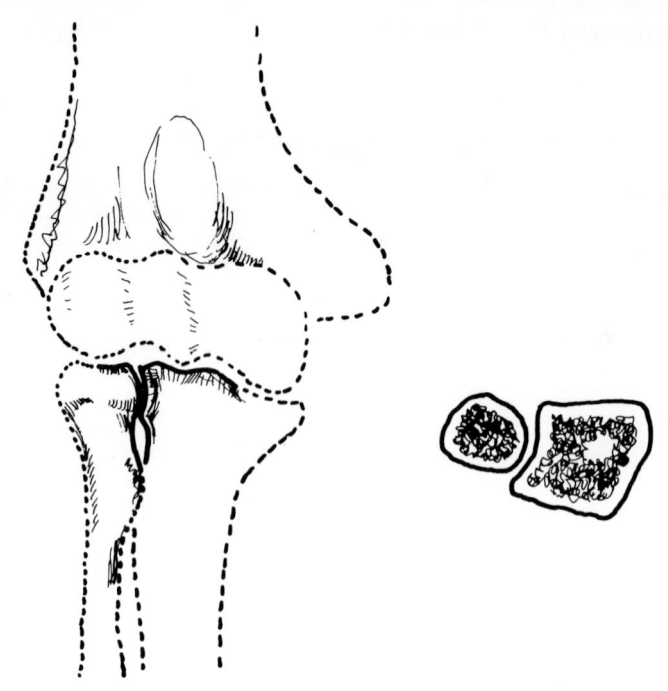

Fig. 1.2f. Pulley (trochoid) joint—superior radio-ulnar joint.

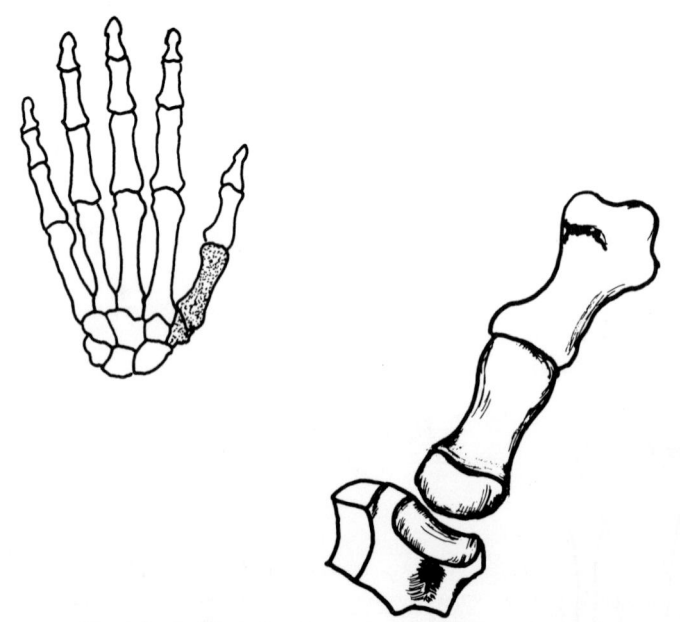

Fig. 1.2g. Saddle (sellar) joint—first carpo-metacarpal joint.

Synovial fluid

This is normally present in only small amounts, and from a knee joint less than ½ml can be extracted. It is a clear, yellow, sticky fluid with a tackiness like that of glycerine and is important for the nutrition of the cartilage as it contains most of the things found in blood plasma. It is also necessary for the lubrication of the joint. One substance peculiar to synovial fluid, not found in the blood, is hyaluronic acid and this is thought to be important in the lubricating mechanism. Lubrication involves both the rubbing of cartilage on cartilage, and of cartilage on the surrounding soft tissue. Some of the proteins in the synovial fluid may also be important for this process. If the synovium becomes inflamed it will produce much more fluid in the joint, so producing a joint effusion. The mechanism is just the same as the production of an effusion in any cavity lined by a membrane (e.g. a pleural effusion over the lung, or a peritoneal effusion in the abdomen).

Capsule

Surrounding and enclosing the whole joint is a capsule of fibrous tissue. The fibres blend into the periosteum of the bone on either side and help to maintain the joint's stability. Certain areas of the capsule may become thickened to form definite ligaments. Other ligaments and tendons may pass close to the joint and so strengthen it. Indeed, in some areas these may become incorporated into the actual joint capsule.

Nerve supply

The capsule and the synovium are supplied with nerve fibres, whereas the articular cartilage is devoid of nervous tissue and is therefore insensitive. A sprain of the joint is painful because it tears the capsule with its abundant nerve supply. In osteoarthrosis there is some instability of the joint, and minor sprains may occur with sudden onset of pain, which subsides as the damage heals. An effusion into the joint may produce pain by distending the sensitive joint capsule.

Blood supply

We have already indicated that the cartilage has no blood supply, relying for its nutrition on the synovial fluid which is pumped in and out of its pores. If no pressure is put on a joint for a long time the cartilage degenerates, because this pumping action does not occur. Conversely, if cartilage is kept under constant pressure it also degenerates because, without intermittent pressure, there cannot be pumping. The synovium, however, has a rich blood supply. It readily becomes inflamed and produces all the signs of inflammation, swelling, heat, redness, tenderness, and painful movement. Involvement of a tendon in disease may alter the position of the joint. Because the tendons slip to one side of the metacarpo-phalangeal joints in rheumatoid arthritis, they pull the fingers into ulnar deviation. In Dupuytren's contracture, thickening of the palmar fascia pulls on the flexor tendons and may produce flexion of the fingers with a benedictus (blessing) sign. Inflammation around a tendon sheath may also prevent a full range of movement at the joint which the tendon serves.

Muscles

The proper functioning of a joint depends not only on the immediate structures but also on the muscles associated with it. An arthritis rapidly produces wasting of associated muscles; the joint is painful and therefore the muscle 'splints' it, rather than moves it. This is often seen in the quadriceps muscle of the thigh, when the knee is affected. After the joint trouble has subsided, the patient may complain that the 'joint lets me down'. This is usually due to muscle weakness, and emphasises the need to build up the muscle by appropriate exercises. In spastic conditions, such as a stroke, spasm of the muscles may hold a joint in flexion (e.g. the hand). If this persists, changes occur in the capsule and a permanent flexion contracture develops. This may also be seen in some paraplegic patients at the knee.

Intra-articular structures

Inside the joint capsule other structures may be found. The cartilage surface may have an additional rim (labrum); this is seen at the hip. Similar margins are present in the shoulder on the glenoid of the scapula. These lips deepen the joint cavity and make the joint more stable. Discs of cartilage may also be found inside the joint. They are called menisci and are frequently torn by footballers. Such discs are also found in the knee, temporo-mandibular, and sometimes the acromio-clavicular joints. They function as shock absorbers, improve the shape of the joint to make it more stable, act as chocks to prevent undue forward gliding of one surface on another, and protect the joint margin by sliding under the joint in certain movements.

Ligaments

These may be incorporated within the joint. Such ligaments, like the cruciate ligaments (so called because they cross over each other from front to back) of the knee, are often surrounded by a sheath of synovial membrane (Fig. 1.3). The bicipital tendon which runs through the shoulder also has a sheath of synovial lining.

Connective tissue

The joint capsule is composed largely of connective tissue; this is widespread throughout the body. Indeed in one form or another it is found in every organ since it is the tissue which holds things together—

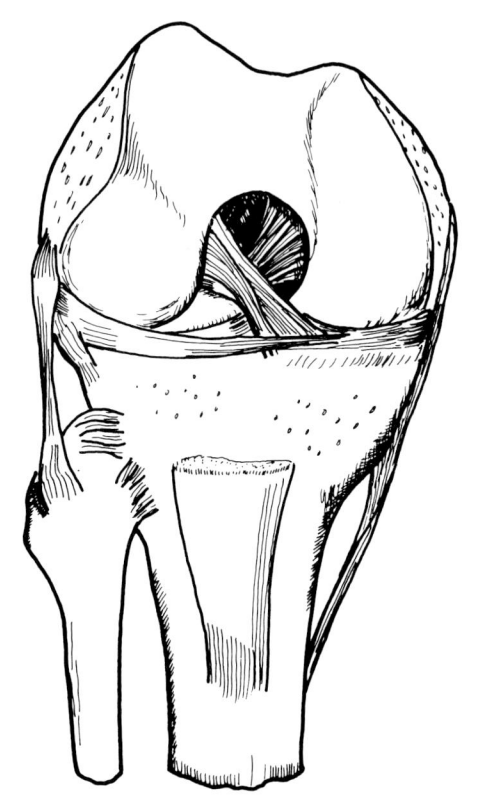

Fig. 1.3. Knee showing cruciate ligaments.

as the name 'connective' suggests. It contains varying amounts of 'collagen' fibres, 'elastin' fibres, and 'ground substance' in between. Where distension is required, elastin predominates as in the walls of larger blood vessels. Where strength is required, collagen predominates as in the joint capsule. Certain disorders which affect the joints, such as rheumatoid arthritis and systemic lupus erythematosus involve this connective tissue widely and are not confined to articular structures. Indeed in some of them the involvement of organs other than joints is the major problem. These diseases have been grouped together under the name 'collagen diseases'. Because we now recognise that the collagen is probably not the part primarily involved, there is a tendency to abandon the term 'collagen diseases' and instead talk of 'connective tissue disorders'. However, it is probably best to be as exact as possible with a specific diagnosis, such as systemic lupus erythematosus, dermatomyositis, systemic sclerosis, scleroderma, or polyarteritis nodosa. Nevertheless, there are overlap cases and the overall term 'connective tissue disorders' has the merit of drawing a common group of diseases together, although it should be noted that profound differences exist between classic cases.

Loads

It is not usually realised that during a normal walking cycle the load on a leg joint can reach over five times body weight, so that loads of about 500-700lb can occur in the hip of a sound person.

The lower loads in the ankle compared with the hip and knee may account for the lower incidence of osteoarthrosis in that joint, and the few symptoms it exhibits. The load varies in a walking cycle. Maximum loads occur at heel strike and toe take-off. The use of a walking stick, because it gives a wider base for the body, may reduce the load on a hip to one and a half times body weight. This explains the value of a stick for patients with osteoarthrosis of the hip, and encouragement should be given to patients who may be reluctant to use what they regard as the badge of crippledom or old age.

The loads on joints vary with different activities. Thus the patello-femoral joint has a greater load in coming down stairs than in ordinary walking, and this is reflected in the difficulty osteoarthrotic patients have with this manoeuvre. Part of the difficulty may also be due to the relation of the centre of gravity of the body to the feet, so that it is more difficult to balance.

Lubrication

A lot of work has been done in recent years on how joints are actually lubricated. It would appear that in various phases of movement, different mechanisms operate. At times a film of synovial fluid separates the surfaces. On other occasions the hyaluronic acid acts by attaching itself loosely to the surface of the cartilage and the layers rub against each other rather like the pile of a carpet. This prevents direct contact and damage. The mechanism is supplemented by a form of lubrication unique to joints. We have termed it 'boosted lubrication' by fluid entrapment and enrichment.

The cartilage surface is surprisingly rough by engineering standards and synovial fluid is trapped in the hollows. Under pressure the watery part of the synovial fluid escapes sideways and some into the cartilage, but the pores are too small to let through the big hyaluronic acid and protein molecules, which are bound to the cartilage surface. They therefore stay behind and enrich the fluid so that at precisely the moment when the joint requires the stickiest lubricant, nature has arranged it so that this is precisely what happens.

2
Rheumatic Diseases in the Community

Prevalence
Rheumatism and Industry
Rheumatism and the National Health Service
Rheumatism and the Home

Prevalence

Rheumatic disorders are extremely common and nearly everyone who reaches the age of 75 is likely to have had some form of rheumatic complaint in his lifetime. This varies, however, from the trivial to the crippling. It strikes without fear or favour and historically Frederick the Great of Prussia had to give up flute playing because of rheumatism in his fingers: Sir William Harvey, the discoverer of the circulation of blood, used to dunk his gouty feet in ice water to soothe them; and some of the most moving music of Mahler, the great composer, was influenced by his knowledge of his impending death from rheumatic heart disease.

The distribution of rheumatic diseases in the community is very different from that of patients referred to hospital. Figures 2.1 and 2.2 show the diagnosis in over 1,000 patients seen in Leigh, Lancashire, compared with those seen at our Rheumatology Outpatient Clinic at Leeds. The commonest group in the community was labelled as undiagnosed, and rheumatoid arthritis accounted for only 10.4%. In the hospital population, however, rheumatoid arthritis was the most frequent diagnosis (59.2%) whereas those undiagnosed amounted to only a small percentage.

Epidemiological studies give us information not only about the distribution of diseases in different areas, but also some clues to causation. If a disease is more prevalent in a certain environment this may enable us to identify the causative agent. A rather unusual example of this is a form of arthritis called Kashin-Beck disease, which occurs in Siberia. It has now been found that this is caused by eating

Rheumatic Diseases in the Community

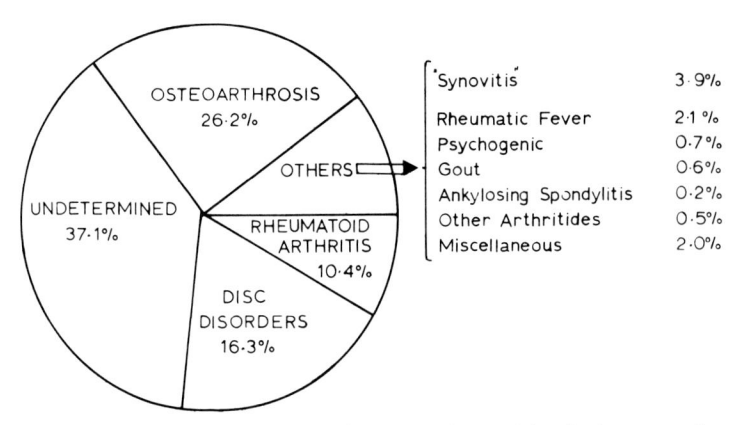

Fig. 2.1. Diagnosis of 1,059 patients with rheumatic complaints in the community.

- Osteoarthrosis 26.2%
- Undetermined 37.1%
- Disc Disorders 16.3%
- Rheumatoid Arthritis 10.4%
- Others:
  - Synovitis 3.9%
  - Rheumatic Fever 2.1%
  - Psychogenic 0.7%
  - Gout 0.6%
  - Ankylosing Spondylitis 0.2%
  - Other Arthritides 0.5%
  - Miscellaneous 2.0%

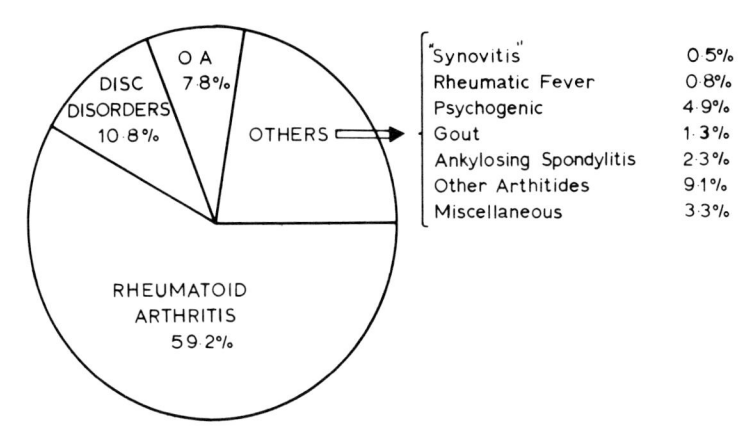

Fig. 2.2. Diagnosis of 1,061 patients attending the Rheumatism Clinic at the Leeds General Infirmary, during a 2-year period.

- OA 7.8%
- Disc Disorders 10.8%
- Rheumatoid Arthritis 59.2%
- Others:
  - Synovitis 0.5%
  - Rheumatic Fever 0.8%
  - Psychogenic 4.9%
  - Gout 1.3%
  - Ankylosing Spondylitis 2.3%
  - Other Arthitides 9.1%
  - Miscellaneous 3.3%

wheat infected by a mould called Fusarium. A more common example would be the high incidence of rheumatic fever in patients who are living in poor and unhygienic home conditions.

Family studies may also be helpful in showing the importance of heredity in disease. It has been shown, for instance, that gout runs in families, as does ankylosing spondylitis. Indeed, recent family studies have shown common links between a number of forms of arthritis that have not been associated previously, such as the arthritis accompanying psoriasis, that accompanying ulcerative colitis, that accompanying Crohn's disease, and that accompanying dysentery and/or non-specific urethritis (a venereal disease).

Some rheumatic diseases are particularly common in certain communities. New Zealand Maori men have a high incidence of gout (10.2%) and some Red Indian tribes in Canada have a high incidence of ankylosing spondylitis. Certain differences may be attributable to social conditions, while others may be due to the sex of the group studied or their age range. Thus ankylosing spondylitis, since it attacks young men predominantly, will be found more frequently in the armed

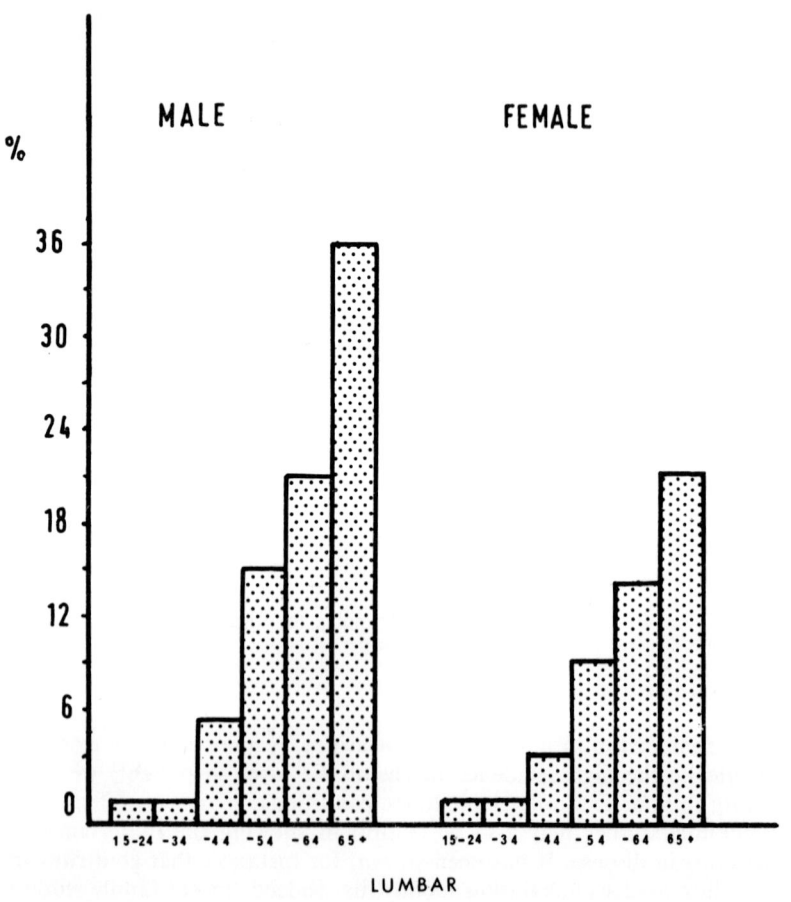

Fig. 2.3a. Prevalence of disc degeneration in Britain related to sex and age: in the lumbar spine.

forces than in the community at large. Again, certain rheumatic diseases were found more commonly in Leigh and Wensleydale than they were in Watford. Since the population of Watford contains many young artisans, the groups are by no means comparable in social structure and the differences were explicable on this basis.

Most rheumatic diseases increase in incidence with advancing years. This is seen strikingly in rheumatoid arthritis where, after the age of 54 years, the incidence becomes 4-5% among men and 15-16% among women.

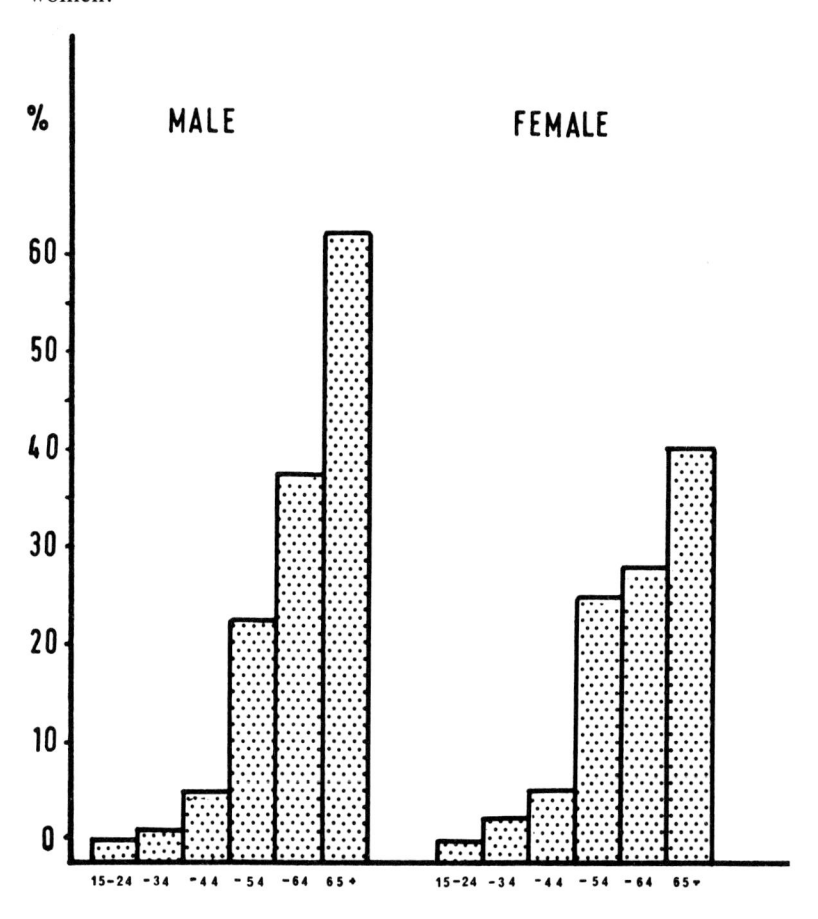

Fig. 2.3b. Prevalence of disc degeneration in Britain related to sex and age: in the cervical spine.

Degeneration in the intervertebral discs of the spine is also more frequent in the older age groups, and moderate to severe changes are very frequent over the age of 65. In the cervical spine such changes occurred in 62% of the men and 41% of the women in that age group. Lumbar disc changes were seen in 47% of the men and 25% of the women over 65 years of age (Fig. 2.3).

The incidence of changes of osteoarthrosis seen on x-ray increases markedly with age, as might be anticipated. It will be seen from Table 2.1 which shows the results of x-raying a sample of the population (not

Age Group (yrs)	% Involved
15—84	51
15—24	11
75+	96

Table 2.1 Radiological survey in community, at least one joint showing osteoarthrosis.

patients coming for medical advice) that as early as 15-24 years a single joint may show some evidence of degeneration in 10% of subjects. The subjects with only one joint involved were equally distributed among the sexes. However, severer forms of disease evidenced by four or more joints involved were found more frequently among women (Table 2.2).

Surveys in the North of England showed that 64% of a random sample of the population who were interviewed had suffered rheumatic symptoms at some time. 35% had some rheumatic complaint at the time of interview, 25% had lost work due to rheumatic complaints and this absence from work had lasted for at least three months in 9% of the total number. Disc degeneration of the spine and osteoarthrosis were the commonest rheumatic diseases keeping men off work, and rheumatoid arthritis was the most frequent cause of women being absent. As far as the more severe forms of rheumatic diseases are concerned, there is little difference in the prevalence over the northern hemisphere. Comparisons of the prevalence of rheumatoid arthritis in England and Jamaica show similar numbers involved in the two

	% Involved	
Age Group (yrs)	Male	Female
15—84	24	36
15—24	0	0
75+	51	75

Table 2.2 Radiological survey in community, four or more joints showing osteoarthrosis.

countries. Fewer Jamaicans had suffered loss of work because of the disease, either because the warmer West Indian climate made the symptoms less troublesome or because the lack of unemployment and sickness benefits encouraged people to stay at work despite their disease.

During this century the occurrence of rheumatic fever in Great Britain has fallen dramatically. This is due to better housing conditions and improved sanitation with a consequent diminution of streptococcal infections. The advent of penicillin has, of course, made some difference, but the major factor producing the drop in incidence is improved public health.

Rheumatism and Industry

Figure 2.4 shows the days lost to industry through various illnesses in the 1950's and it will be seen that the rheumatic diseases headed the list. Still, in 1973, days lost from work due to rheumatic complaints

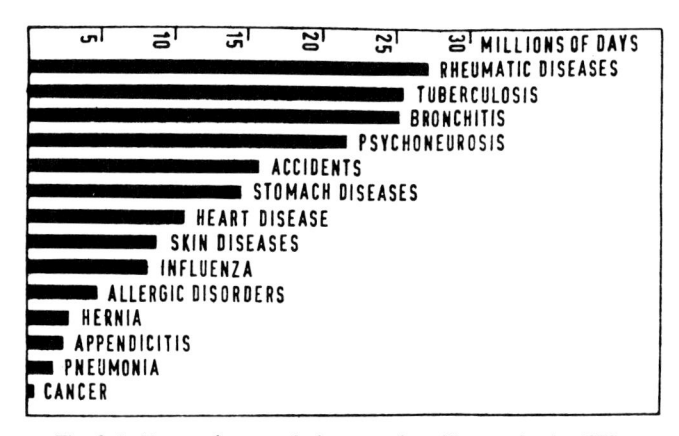

```
                                         MILLIONS OF DAYS
         5    10   15   20   25   30
                                         RHEUMATIC DISEASES
                                         TUBERCULOSIS
                                         BRONCHITIS
                                         PSYCHONEUROSIS
                                         ACCIDENTS
                                         STOMACH DISEASES
                                         HEART DISEASE
                                         SKIN DISEASES
                                         INFLUENZA
                                         ALLERGIC DISORDERS
                                         HERNIA
                                         APPENDICITIS
                                         PNEUMONIA
                                         CANCER
```

Fig. 2.4. Absence from work due to various illnesses in the 1950s.

rank as second only to those lost from respiratory diseases. In 1955 three quarters of a million patients claimed sickness benefit because of rheumatic diseases and 27 million working days were lost, equivalent to £32 million in wages. A total of 37.5 million days were lost due to these diseases in the UK between 1970 and 1971. The magnitude of this problem is such that if strikes, which produced 10.9 million days lost in 1970/71, are a danger to the economy, then rheumatic disorders are a disaster.

It is difficult to obtain precise information from such a breakdown because of the poor categorisation. It will be noted, however, that complaints related to the back are prominent.

A detailed survey of rheumatic complaints among men in industry showed that back pain accounted for 50% of all such diseases and 60% of the time lost. Certain groups of workers are more prone to develop rheumatic complaints than others, and this is well shown in Fig. 2.5. Much of this disability is due to poor working

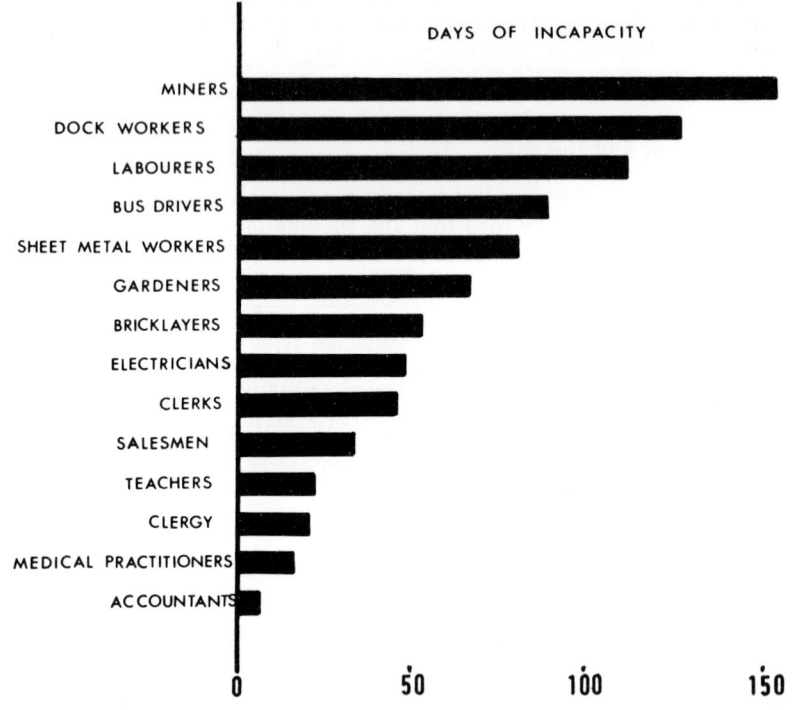

Fig. 2.5. Days of incapacity from arthritis and rheumatism lost per 100 men at risk in the United Kingdom during the year ended June 1962.

conditions and is preventable. Thus, the design of a capstan lathe is such that the ideal operator would be a man four feet tall with an arm span of over eight feet!

Miners get trouble with their knees called 'beat knee' due to a mixture of injury and infection. Workers with compressed air develop Caisson disease due to aseptic necrosis of the bone and cartilage caused by bubbles of nitrogen circulating in the blood. This results in osteoarthrosis. Moulders in iron foundries, who have to adopt abnormal postures while exerting severe physical effort, have a high incidence of disc problems in the back and pneumatic drillers are said to develop osteoarthrosis of the elbows.

The smallest number of new cases occurs among professional people and the most among unskilled workers. This applies to all rheumatic diseases except gout and is not entirely explicable on the basis of the extra trauma of normal work.

As a reason for patients being on the Handicapped Register the rheumatic complaints assume increasing importance with advancing age, so that between the ages of 50 and 65 years, 25% of such patients are suffering from rheumatic disorders.

Rheumatism and the National Health Service

In the General Infirmary at Leeds in 1974 rheumatological new patients comprised 7.5% of all medical out-patients and in-patients. In terms of National Health Service expenditure, in 1968 £28 millions were spent on hospital services and £16.3 millions on domiciliary services, making a total of £44.3 millions devoted to rheumatic diseases. The expenditure on surgical shoes alone amounted to £1.2 million in that year.

Rheumatism and the Home

Quite apart from the number of days lost from work, a good deal of disability is found in the home. Of three million people impaired to some degree with rheumatic complaints, one million are being handicapped by their impairment. Of these, two-thirds were over the age of 65 and two-thirds were women. Amongst the elderly 40% of all handicap is due to arthritis. The rheumatic diseases may also aggravate the problems that face elderly people who may be disabled from other conditions.

A study in the Isle of Wight has shown that, compared with other disabilities, sufferers from rheumatoid arthritis are more likely to be confined to their homes. The problem is heightened when the patient is living alone. All our patients suffering from rheumatic diseases who are admitted to hospital and some of the out-patients have a full assessment in the activities of daily living by the occupational therapist and the majority require assistance in some way or another to cope with their household tasks. Careful analysis has to be made of toilet facilities and domestic duties. For any disabled person independence in toilet is of vital importance and mobility is a very important factor in their life pattern.

Cooking is often a problem and difficulty in preparing meals may well explain why a recent survey of ours has shown that the majority of patients with rheumatoid arthritis have a deficient calcium intake. Special gadgets may be needed to help with dressing with washing and with the use of the lavatory. Other problems may be experienced in sexual activity and a study by Professor Harry Currey at the London Hospital has revealed how common this is. Many of these patients desire advice about this subject, but it has been found that most preferred it to be by booklet rather than direct discussion. A booklet has, therefore been prepared.* In a recent study of ours in which we have looked at young married women with rheumatoid arthritis, we have observed the impact on the husband and the effect on inter-relationships in the family. It is apparent that a good deal more explanation is often required to the spouse as well as to the sufferer about the patient's condition.

Relatively simple limitations may pose considerable problems to rheumatic sufferers—for example, inability to cut the toenails was a prominent problem in the Isle of Wight survey. Of 100 consecutive patients whom we have looked at from this point of view, we found that 49% required chiropody. Sometimes this was due to an inability to reach the feet, sometimes to a weakness of the hands and at other times due to specific problems, such as callosities under the metatarsal heads.

The problems posed to the community by rheumatic diseases are enormous both in extent and expense. Recent measures such as the introduction of a register of handicapped persons, and mortality trends which enable an increasing number of patients to live into their seventh and eighth decades are all serving to increase awareness of the enormous social burden the rheumatic diseases place on the community.

*'Marriage, Sex and Arthritis' prepared by the Arthritis and Rheumatism Council in collaboration with Dr Wendy Greengross.

3
Rheumatoid Arthritis

Definition
Aetiology
Pathology
Clinical Findings
Course of the Disease
The Rheumatoid Hand
Other Joints
Extra-articular Manifestations
Juvenile Chronic Arthritis
Investigations
Treatment
Prognosis

Rheumatoid arthritis is the disease which most people identify with the subject of rheumatology. In terms of the total number of people with rheumatic diseases, the proportion suffering from rheumatoid arthritis is not high, but because of the nature, duration and possible severity of this disease it forms a large part of the 'rheumatology' seen in hospitals. In the Rheumatism Clinic at Leeds 52% of the out-patients seen suffer from rheumatoid arthritis. It is more prevalent in older women (Fig. 3.1).

Rheumatoid arthritis deserves close study and scrupulous attention to detail by all types of staff involved in its management. Details which appear insignificant to the casual observer may be crucial to achieving much good, or producing great harm, to the rheumatoid patient.

Definition

Rheumatoid arthritis is a chronic inflammatory disease of unknown cause. The major part of the disease is suffered by the joints which are involved in a symmetrical fashion with the small peripheral joints being most affected. There is also a marked systemic part of the disease which can affect many organs other than joints throughout the body (sometimes called 'extra-articular manifestations'). Subcutaneous nodules which are diagnostic of the disease occur in 17-25% of our patients with rheumatoid arthritis. The amount of inflammation occurring tends to wax and wane spontaneously, and incomplete forms are common. The majority of patients give positive agglutination tests for rheumatoid factor (see page 187) in their blood.

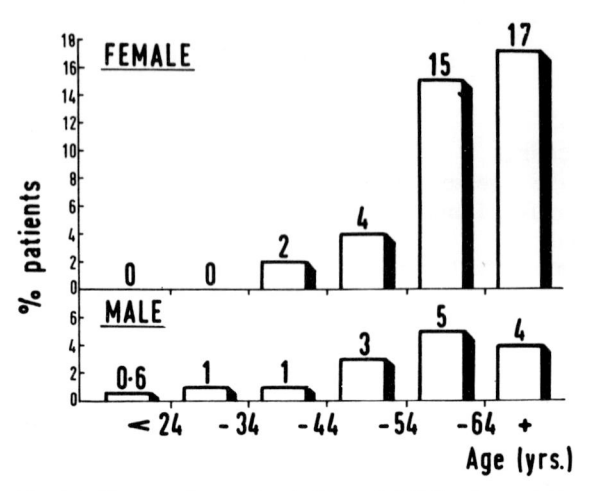

Fig. 3.1. The prevalence of probable and definite rheumatoid arthritis related to age.

Aetiology

The cause of rheumatoid arthritis is unknown. It may start at any time from childhood to old age, but the peak age of onset is in the 40-50 age group (Fig. 3.2). Women are affected more often than men. In the general population the sex ratio of female:male is 3:2, but in a rheumatic clinic it is 3:1. The disease often appears to start after some physical or emotional stress. In spite of popular belief rheumatoid arthritis is not found only in cool, damp climates. For example, the disease is found as often in Jamaica as in England, and the only country that is entirely spared is Tristan da Cunha.

There are at present two main theories as to the cause of rheumatoid arthritis. The suggestion that the disease is an infection was first made in the last century, and many patients lost their teeth and tonsils as the physician searched for hidden foci of infection. It has recently been revived by claims that two classes of organisms, diphtheroids and mycoplasma, have been found in patients with rheumatoid arthritis. These findings are, however, not very consistent. The second major

Rheumatoid Arthritis

theory is that of auto-immunity. The immune system of the body is designed to protect the body from outside invasion. In order to do this, it has to be able to distinguish between the body itself and the outside invader, or the defence mechanisms could be turned on a part of the body. It has been suggested that this distinction between 'self' and 'not self' fails in rheumatoid arthritis, and the body embarks on a self-

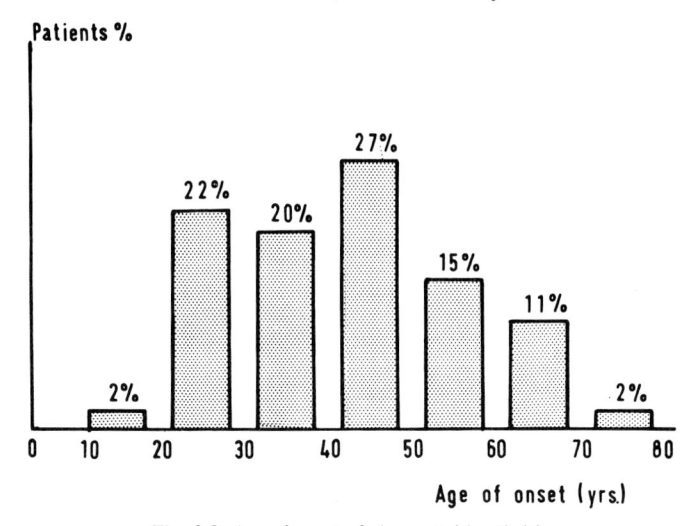

Fig. 3.2. Age of onset of rheumatoid arthritis.

destructive path. While there is ample evidence that the immune system of the body behaves abnormally during the course of rheumatoid arthritis, it is not as yet clear that this is a self-initiated process and thus truly 'auto-immune'. Research into these theories of causation is, however, hampered by the fact that rheumatoid arthritis does not occur in animals, nor can it be produced in them.

There is a little evidence that heredity may play a role, but this is not at all clear. Because the disease is fairly common after the age of 40 it would not be surprising to find another relative with it by chance. Hormonal factors may also have some part to play. The disease goes into remission in pregnancy (an observation which led Hench to use cortisone in rheumatoid arthritis), recurring after the baby is born. Sometimes it begins after childbirth, or is closely connected with the menopause.

Pathology

Rheumatoid arthritis is essentially a synovitis—i.e. it produces inflammation of the lining of the joint, the synovium. The first changes are hyperaemia (increase in blood flow and dilatation of blood vessels), oedema, infiltration by inflammatory cells (white blood cells) and the production of an exudate rich in fibrin on the cell surface. As the disease progresses the synovial tissue becomes thicker and more engorged. The inflamed tissue spreads in a sinister film across the surface of the joint cartilage, where it is called *pannus*. Underneath this pannus the cartilage is destroyed, and eventually the pannus may cause destruction of the underlying bone. This destructive process produces the erosions that are seen on x-ray. The over-production of an abnormal synovial fluid by the inflamed synovial tissue continues, and the joint may become swollen because of the increased amount of both tissue and fluid present. When the inflammation decreases the joint may be permanently lax because of irreversible stretching of the surrounding tissues which has taken place, or the disturbed architecture resulting from the destruction of cartilage and bone.

Clinical Findings

The clinical signs are those expected in the presence of inflammation. The joint may be painful, hot, red and swollen and function is decreased. The swelling is of a soft-tissue nature, in contrast to the bony swelling of osteoarthrosis. In addition, profound stiffness, especially on first wakening in the morning, is a characteristic complaint of patients with rheumatoid arthritis in an active phase. As the disease settles, the duration and severity of the morning stiffness decreases. At a later stage laxity and deformity of the joints may be seen which may persist after all signs of active inflammation have subsided.

Course of the Disease

Rheumatoid arthritis may start as an acute illness, with inflammation of many joints, high temperature, sweating and general malaise, but most patients have a more insidious onset of disease. They may notice mild aching in the joints, stiffness, especially in the morning, or a general feeling of tiredness often accompanied by loss of appetite and weight. Many present to their doctors because they feel 'rundown' or 'out of sorts', and it is only on careful questioning that the joint symptoms may be mentioned.

The course of rheumatoid arthritis is one of exacerbations and remissions, that is there are times of exacerbation when the inflammation is active—the 'flare-up'—and times of remission when there is little or no inflammation taking place. The patient may still have symptoms and signs during the phase of remission because of damage that has taken place in the past.

The Rheumatoid Hand

The hand has been described as 'the arthritic patient's calling card'. The pattern of disease there is easily noticed, both by the patient and the nurse. It provides a strong clue to the diagnosis, and it may cause a great deal of the patient's disability. The joints particularly involved are the proximal interphalangeal (p.i.p.) joints and the metacarpo-phalangeal (m.c.p.) joints, especially those of the index and middle fingers. The contrast of hand joints involved by rheumatoid arthritis and osteoarthrosis is shown in Fig. 3.3. The swelling of these joints may

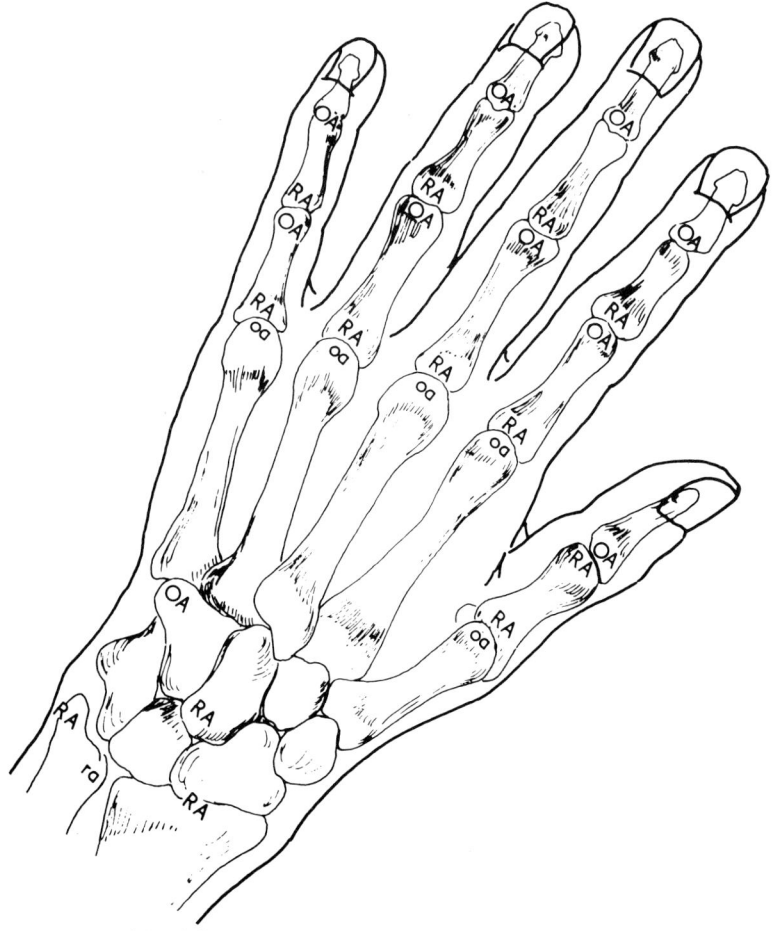

Fig. 3.3. The joints of the hand predominantly affected by rheumatoid arthritis and osteoarthrosis.

be accentuated by wasting of the small muscles in the hand, giving it a shrivelled appearance. The fingers tend to drift towards the ulnar border of the hand (ulnar deviation) from the m.c.p. joints (Fig. 3.4). This deviation is usually most marked in the little finger, and involves each successive finger to a lesser degree. Two other typical deformities of the fingers which may occur are the swan-neck in which the p.i.p.

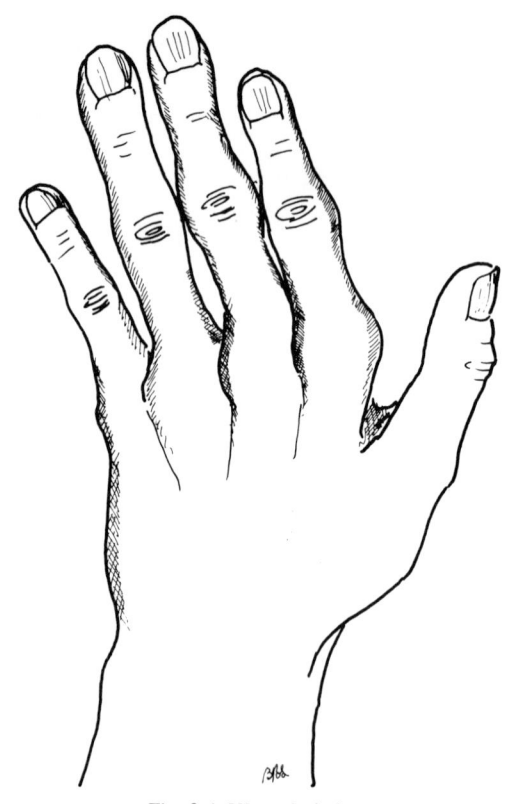

Fig. 3.4. Ulnar deviation.

joint is hyperextended and the distal interphalangeal (d.i.p.) joint flexed, and the boutonniere in which the p.i.p. joint is fixed in flexion and the d.i.p. hyperextended. The most important feature of the rheumatoid hand is its function, not its appearance. Function may be assessed either as part of an examination or by the observation of the patient's limitation in such everyday tasks as washing or eating. The usual major difficulty is in flexion of the fingers, especially when the m.c.p. joints become subluxed.

The wrist is often involved early in rheumatoid arthritis. The lowest part of the ulna, the ulnar styloid, often has an overlying swelling and is tender. Later it may be prominent because the radio-ulnar joint subluxes, and at this point the 'piano-key sign' may be observed, in which the lower end of the ulna may be pressed down like a springy piano note (with a not very musical sound coming from the patient's mouth). The radio-carpal joint and the joints in the wrist may also be involved. Hand and wrist joint involvement must be considered together as the extensor tendons of the fingers cross the wrist and may be inhibited by inflammation there.

Other Joints

The toes are frequently involved early in the course of rheumatoid arthritis, especially the metatarso-phalangeal (m.t.p.) joints. The phalanges tend to 'ride up' on the metatarsal heads, the toes becoming clawed. Weight-bearing then takes place on the metatarsal heads which is very painful. Callosities, which are painful in themselves, tend to form under the prominent bones, and the toes tend to rub on shoes and become painful and ulcerated. The toes may also drift into fibular deviation as the fingers do into ulnar deviation.

All the other synovial joints in the body may become involved by rheumatoid arthritis. Great disability arises from involvement of the knees. The position of greatest comfort when the knees are painful is to be with them flexed. To facilitate this, patients or well-meaning nurses may put a pillow under the knees. This cannot be too strongly condemned, as it may lead to permanent flexion deformities. Laxity of the ligaments of the knee produced by swelling is also important, as severe varus (bow-leg) or valgus (knock-knee) deformities may be produced.

Ankle and subtaloid joint involvement may produce intractable problems, the feet tending to evert with the body weight increasing this everting force. Hip joint involvement may also cause pain and difficulty in walking, though the outward signs of inflammation may be less obvious because the joint is deeply seated. Secondary osteoarthrosis may occur in any joint deformed by rheumatoid inflammation, but occurs particularly in the hip.

In the upper limb, shoulder joint involvement may reduce the ability to elevate the arms and cause problems with tasks such as hair combing. Damage to the elbow may produce flexion deformities and an inability to rotate the forearm. Neck movements may be painful and restricted. Subluxation of the atlanto-axial joint (between the first and second cervical vertebrae) may occur and may cause compression on the spinal cord with occasional development of quadriplegia and sudden death.

Extra-articular Manifestations

It cannot be too strongly stressed that organs other than joints are involved in rheumatoid arthritis and for this reason some authorities prefer the name rheumatoid *disease* to rheumatoid *arthritis* as they feel that it highlights the generalised nature of the condition. Tendon sheaths are frequently affected, and much of the swelling on the dorsum of the wrist may come from the tendon sheaths of the finger extensor muscles rather than from the wrist joint itself. The tendon itself may rupture, causing 'dropped fingers' requiring surgical repair. Nodules in the tendon sheath may interfere with the smooth running of the tendon. In 'trigger finger' the finger can be flexed but the nodules interfere with extension. The finger can, however, be extended by pulling on it, snapping back into position like the trigger of a gun.

Muscles become wasted not only from disease but also from inflammation in them. Quadriceps wasting is often prominent, especially when the knees are swollen. There appears to be a reflex inhibition of the quadriceps caused by the presence of an effusion, and no amount of physiotherapy will increase their bulk under these circumstances.

Subcutaneous rheumatoid nodules are pathognomonic of rheumatoid arthritis; that is they occur in no other disease. They are frequently found at the elbow, but may occur over any bony prominence in the body. Nodules may become ulcerated, usually following injury to them. A particularly awkward site for nodules is in the buttocks over the ischial tuberosities. Ulceration is frequent at this site. Pericarditis occurs in about one third of patients with rheumatoid arthritis, though it rarely causes serious symptoms. Pleurisy and pleural effusion may also occur, and fibrosis of the lungs is a less common problem.

Some of the most serious consequences of rheumatoid arthritis arise when vasculitis, or inflammation of the walls of the blood vessels, occurs. This can sometimes be detected clinically by the observation of small black specks at the nail base. These are small areas of dead tissue (infarcts). Ulceration may also be caused by vasculitis and large leg ulcers may be difficult to heal. More seriously, the vasculitis may affect the blood supply to nerves causing a peripheral neuropathy. Nerves may also be involved when pressure occurs in such sites as the tight carpal tunnel when the available space is filled by inflamed synovium.

Involvement of the eyes may also be a serious part of rheumatoid disease. Episcleritis is inflammation in the outer part of the eye, and in juvenile chronic arthritis a band of inflammation—band keratitis— may spread across the cornea causing blindness. Tear secretion may dry up (keratoconjunctivitis sicca) and artificial tears must be prescribed otherwise small specks of dirt fail to be washed away, the cornea becomes scratched and the patient may go blind. Amyloidosis, a

Rheumatoid Arthritis

condition where an abnormal protein called amyloid is deposited in widespread sites throughout the body, may be caused by rheumatoid arthritis. The extra-articular part of rheumatoid arthritis is attracting greater attention among doctors at present. Its importance to the nurse is the constant awareness that patients with rheumatoid arthritis have a generalised illness, not just a disease of their joints.

Juvenile Chronic Arthritis

Polyarthritis in children is often called 'Still's disease' but it is now realised that this is a collection of diseases rather than one only. The joints involved at the onset are shown in Fig. 3.5. Some children go on to develop adult rheumatoid arthritis and others adult ankylosing spondylitis. True Still's disease may present with a high temperature, enlarged lymph glands or a large spleen. A transient rash may be seen during episodes of pyrexia only, fading as the temperature returns to normal. The pyrexia often responds to salicylate therapy. The frequency of features outside the joints is shown in Fig. 3.6. Interference with growth occurs when inflammation is at the growing bone end, and the epiphyses involved fuse early with consequent stunting of

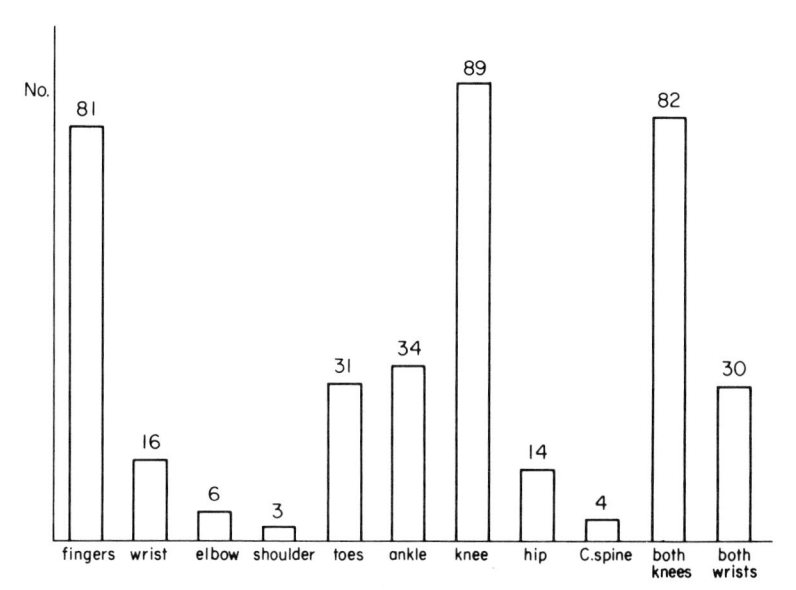

Fig. 3.5. Joints involved at the onset of Still's disease in 544 patients from Scandinavia.

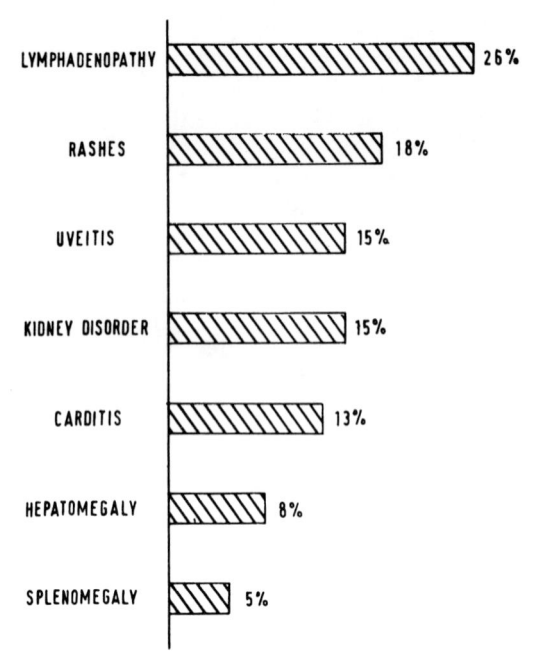

Feature	Percentage
LYMPHADENOPATHY	26%
RASHES	18%
UVEITIS	15%
KIDNEY DISORDER	15%
CARDITIS	13%
HEPATOMEGALY	8%
SPLENOMEGALY	5%

Fig. 3.6. Extra-articular features of Still's disease in 151 patients.

growth. In the jaw it produces a small receding jaw (micrognathism), giving a profile sometimes known as bird facies or shrewmouse profile (Fig. 3.7). Growth may also be stunted when daily corticosteroids are given, but equivalent doses given on alternate days allow normal growth to take place.

The outlook for patients with Still's disease is good on the whole. For example, a follow-up study of 105 patients undertaken 15 years after they had been treated at Taplow Hospital showed that 73 were able to get to work on foot or by public transport, 27 used their own cars, 5 had invalid cars and only 2 required other special arrangements.

Investigations

The most specific diagnostic blood test for rheumatoid arthritis is detection of rheumatoid factor, an abnormal protein complex, in the blood. This is usually carried out using a sheep cell agglutination test (SCAT). Using this test, 80% of patients with rheumatoid arthritis are SCAT positive, although positive tests may also be found in 5% of the

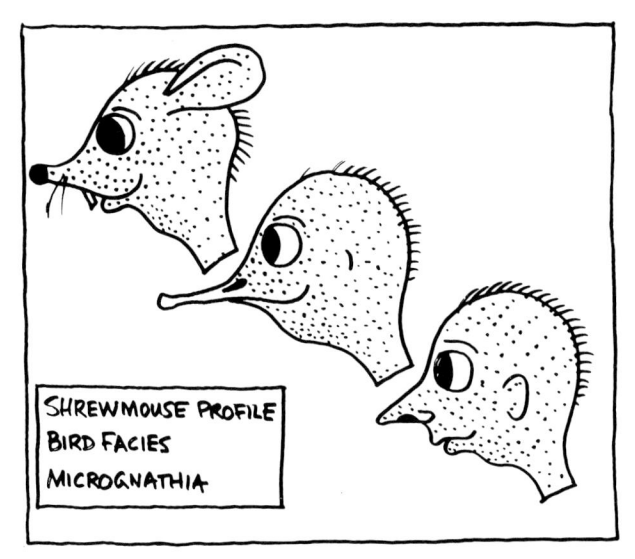

Fig. 3.7. Micrognathia of Still's disease—sometimes called shrew-mouse profile or bird facies. (By courtesy of Dr John Moll.)

normal population. The extent and severity of the inflammation going on at any time can be assessed by measuring the ESR, although this can be affected by a wide variety of other conditions. Anaemia is very common in rheumatoid arthritis. It is usually the 'anaemia of chronic disease' rather than iron deficient. Over the long term a good picture of the progression of the disease may be obtained from looking at serial haemoglobin levels. Plasma proteins may also be disturbed by the inflammatory process with the globulin level rising and the albumin sometimes falling.

X-rays are valuable both in the diagnosis of rheumatoid arthritis and in following the extent of joint damage. There are four radiological changes (Fig. 3.8). Bone loss around the joints, juxta-articular osteoporosis, is seen early in the course of the disease. Osteoporosis may later become more widespread, especially where corticosteroids are used in treatment. The next change seen is loss of joint space. This dark gap between the bone ends is not in fact a space, but represents the articular cartilage which lets the x-rays through. Narrowing of this gap, therefore, shows the extent of cartilage loss. Erosions are produced by destruction of the cartilage and subsequently bone under the pannus, which creeps in from the joint margin. Thus they are usually seen first at the edge of the joint (marginal erosions) but may also appear in the middle of the joint (central erosions). Finally, the x-ray will show subluxation or dis-

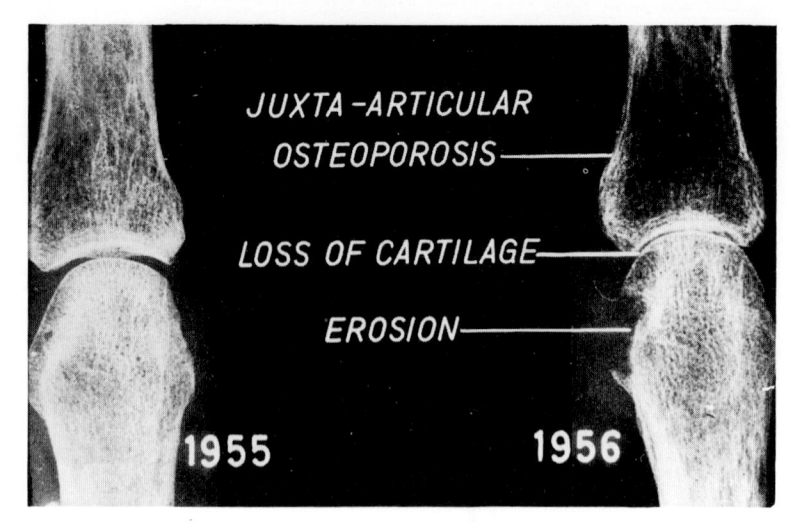

Fig. 3.8. Progress of x-ray changes in a rheumatoid joint over one year.

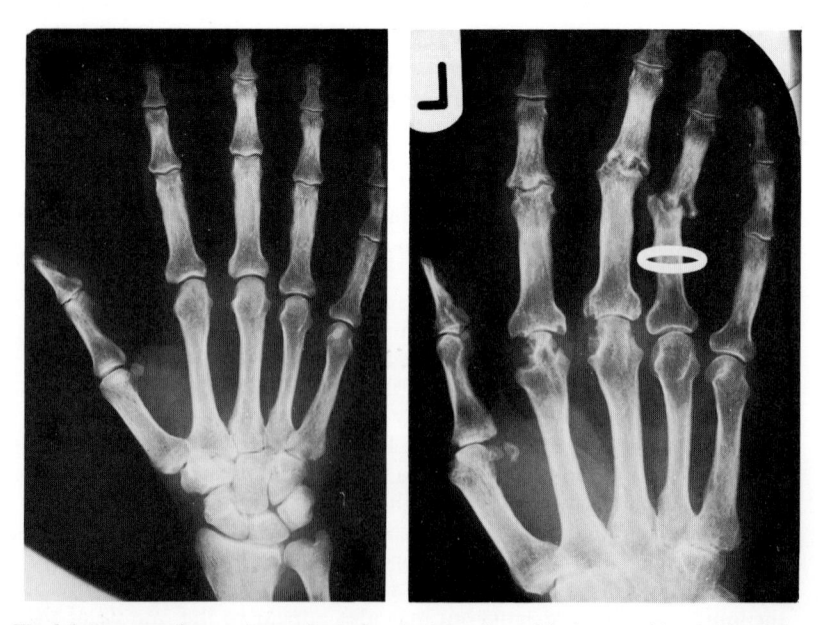

Fig. 3.9. Progress of x-ray changes in the hands of a patient with rheumatoid arthritis. A) At beginning of disease. B) 8 years later.

location of the joints and other gross abnormalities such as gross distortion of bone architecture (Fig. 3.9).

Treatment

The term 'management' is more appropriate in rheumatoid arthritis as there is as yet no form of treatment leading to a cure. The basis of therapy is the use of a multi-disciplinary team involving, among others, general practitioners, rheumatologists, orthopaedic surgeons, home and hospital nurses, occupational therapists, physiotherapists, social workers, the disablement resettlement officer (DRO) and voluntary organisations. Each of these aspects are considered in detail elsewhere, but some principles must be stressed with particular respect to the patient with rheumatoid arthritis.

Medical treatment is only effective if the doctor and the patient are able to communicate freely and meaningfully. Patients require unhurried and repeated explanations regarding the consequences of their disease and the means of treating it. The physician must have a wide knowledge of the potential limitations and dangers of the increasing number of available drugs. Combined rheumatic-orthopaedic clinics are now an essential part of the management of the rheumatoid patient and combined in-patient management is essential pre- and postoperatively.

Nurses must have a wide knowledge of the toxic effects of drugs, particularly those such as gold which she is more likely to administer than the doctor. Good basic nursing care is possibly of more importance on a rheumatological ward than any other in the hospital. The alliance of painful, tender joints to fragile skin requires great skill in nursing care. Bed position is vital if flexion deformities are to be prevented. Finally, the nurse is often the patient's confidant and is told the many worries which the patient suffers. In particular, female patients often ask the advice of nurses, rather than doctors, about many domestic and sexual problems which accompany rheumatoid arthritis.

Occupational therapists play a big role in the assessment of patients in activities of daily living and the provision of appropriate modifications to clothing, home or place of work. The support of a social worker or, in our experience more appropriately, a health visitor is needed when the patient returns home. The temperament of physiotherapists treating patients with rheumatoid arthritis needs to be calm and phlegmatic, as progress of these patients is less rapid and dramatic than in many of the situations, such as orthopaedic surgery, in which they work.

Finally, the efforts of all these diverse groups must be co-ordinated, and this is one of the most important aspects of the rheumatologist's care of patients with rheumatoid arthritis.

Prognosis

The degree of disability which a patient will suffer as a result of rheumatoid arthritis cannot be predicted in individual patients. When Dr Bremner of Leeds did a survey in Wensleydale some patients had rheumatoid arthritis of such mild degree they had not even bothered to consult their family doctor, let alone a specialist. Even those patients with disease sufficiently severe to be admitted to hospital may clear up with little disability—indeed 50% have little trouble thereafter (Fig. 3.10). In general, it is important to stress the possibility of little or no handicap occurring, as the diagnosis 'rheumatoid arthritis' means to

THE PROGNOSIS OF RHEUMATOID ARTHRITIS

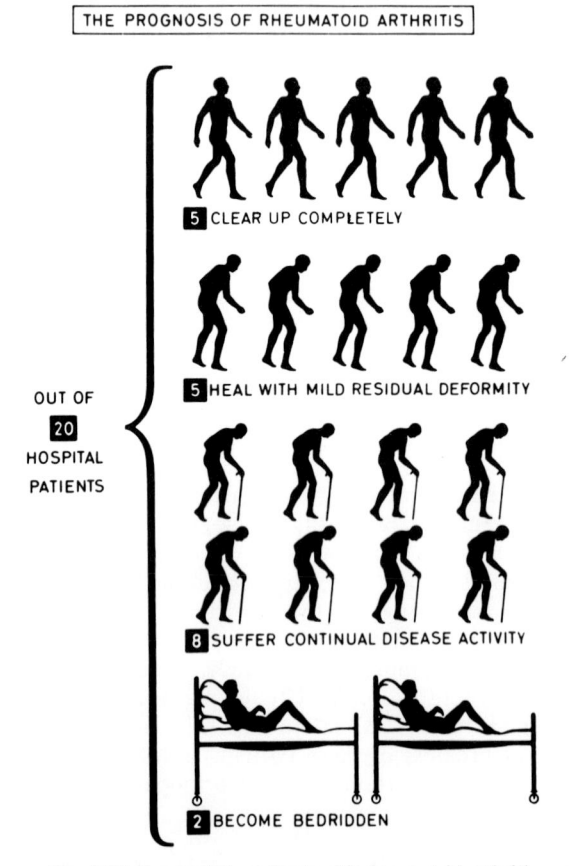

OUT OF 20 HOSPITAL PATIENTS

5 CLEAR UP COMPLETELY

5 HEAL WITH MILD RESIDUAL DEFORMITY

8 SUFFER CONTINUAL DISEASE ACTIVITY

2 BECOME BEDRIDDEN

Fig. 3.10. Prognosis in patients with rheumatoid arthritis sufficiently severe to be admitted to hospital.

many people that they will be permanently crippled. The amount of eventual handicap suffered is influenced by the quality of the care given during acute exacerbations of the disease. In particular, attention to details such as bed position and appropriate splintage is of great importance in the long term. Occasionally rheumatoid arthritis may contribute to the death of the patient, e.g. from heart disease, kidney disease, infection or atlanto-axial subluxation. Sometimes the side effects of treatment may also be fatal.

4
Osteoarthrosis

Types of Osteoarthrosis
Pathology
Clinical Signs
Primary Osteoarthrosis
Secondary Osteoarthrosis
Radiology
Treatment
Surgery

Osteoarthrosis is the disease of the pathological wear in joints. The name osteoarthr*osis* is now preferred to the old term osteoarthr*itis*, as the latter ending implies that there is an inflammatory cause for the condition (as in appendic*itis* or tonsill*itis*). The older term is still used by some people, and others call this condition 'degenerative joint disease'. All three are different names for the same condition. It is a very common form of joint disease, particularly in the elderly, as the results from a thousand post-mortem examinations show (Fig. 4.1).

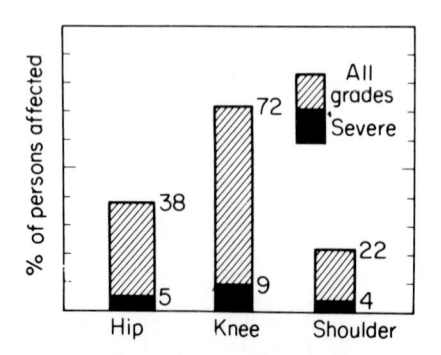

Fig. 4.1. Prevalence of osteoarthrosis data from 1,000 hospital post-mortems.

Types of Osteoarthrosis

There are two types of osteoarthrosis—primary and secondary. Primary osteoarthrosis may occur in one joint only, but usually involves many joints. It is called an idiopathic disease, that is one for which there is no known cause. Secondary osteoarthrosis frequently involves one joint only, and there is an obvious predisposing cause for the condition.

Pathology

The pathology of both types of osteoarthrosis is the same. The first process that can be seen is irregularity of the surface of articular cartilage. This is known as fibrillation of the articular surface. This irregularity increases in depth and eventually cracks and fissures may be seen. At the same time the underlying bone becomes more dense, or sclerotic, and projections called osteophytes grow out from the edges of the joint (Fig. 4.2). These osteophytes are initially composed of cartilage which then ossifies. The formation of osteophytes has been called an attempt by the joint to increase its surface and thus spread the load and decrease the further damage. The process of articular cartilage destruction may continue until the underlying bone is exposed. This may then become smooth, thick and polished, a process known as

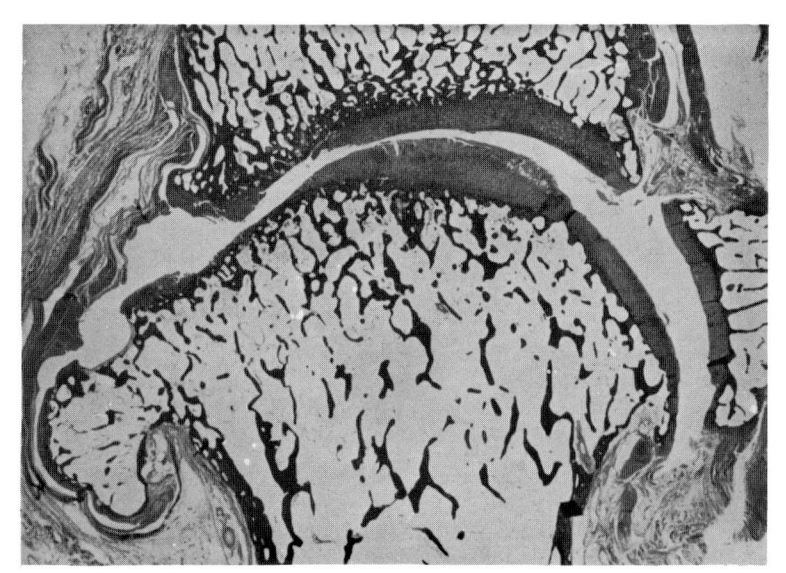

Fig. 4.2. Cross-section of a joint with osteoarthrosis, showing loss of cartilage and marginal osteophyte.

eburnation. Loose fragments of cartilage or bone may flake off into the joint, and these may cause a synovitis. This makes a sharp contrast with the pathological changes in rheumatoid arthritis. In that disease the primary pathological change is inflammation of the synovium (synovitis) with secondary changes in the cartilage and bone. In osteoarthrosis the primary changes are in the cartilage and bone, any synovitis occurring late in the course of the disease and having little effect on its progress.

Clinical Signs

The clinical signs are pain, bony swelling and decreased function in the involved joints. The sequence of events usually starts with a stage of painful swelling at which time there may be some redness and inflammation. The pain subsides, but the bony swelling caused by osteophyte formation remains. The appearance of the joint frequently suffers more than the function. Crepitus or grating may occur as the two irregular articular cartilage surfaces rub together. There is an increased secretion of synovial fluid which is thinner than usual, though not as thin as that which is found in rheumatoid arthritis. The normal lubrication of the joint relies on the articular surfaces being smooth and undulating and the synovial fluid being thick. In osteoarthrosis, the surfaces become rougher and the fluid thinner. The joints therefore 'run rough' accounting for their weakness and their poor function. Further episodes of acute pain and swelling may occur which are probably due to sprains taking place in the unstable joint. The acute episodes settle, but progressive damage may be occurring. Occasionally 'locking' of joints may occur due to the presence of bony or cartilaginous loose bodies in the joints. The type of pain that the patients suffer has been studied particularly in connection with osteoarthrosis of the knees. It was found that three types of pain occurred:
1. muscular (rare)
2. venous—constant deep aching, often at night
3. ligamentous—sharp pain on weightbearing.

Varicose veins are commoner in patients with osteoarthrosis than in other patients attending hospital and patients with varicosities are more likely to suffer from the venous type of pain.

Primary Osteoarthrosis

Primary osteoarthrosis is much commoner in women than in men. It usually occurs after the age of 40 years and is often associated with the menopause (Fig. 4.3). At one time it was the custom to describe these patients as having a special type of arthritis which was named 'menopausal arthritis', but this is now known to be generalised osteoarthrosis. Generalised osteoarthrosis may involve almost any joint in the body, but the pattern of involvement (Fig. 4.4) contrasts with that in rheumatoid arthritis. The joints most commonly involved are

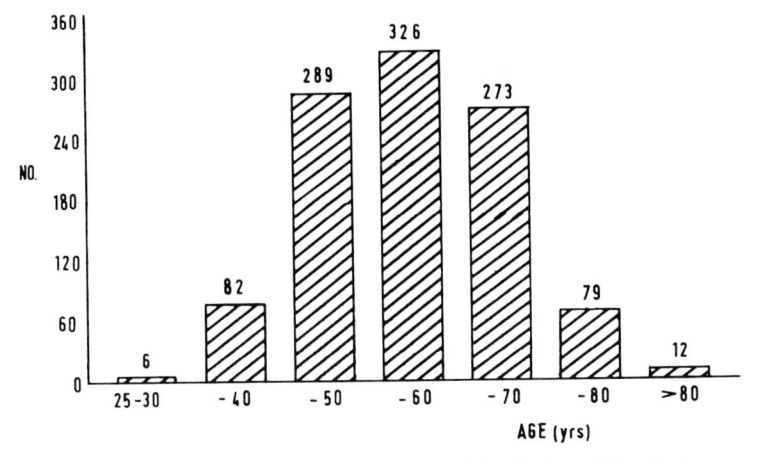

Fig. 4.3. The age of onset of osteoarthrosis of the hip in 1,067 patients.

the distal interphalangeal (d.i.p.) joints. Bony swelling of the proximal interphalangeal joints may also occur (Bouchard's nodes) and a thickening of the tissue over the dorsum of that joint may form a Garrod's pad (Fig. 4.5). The hard bony swelling of the joints contrasts with the soft, synovial swelling of the proximal interphalangeal joints in rheumatoid arthritis. It is important to make this clear differentiation to the patients, as many people think that the development of swelling of the finger joints means that they have rheumatoid arthritis and will therefore become crippled. They are often very relieved to be told the true diagnosis and good prognosis. The d.i.p. joints often have small hard lumps, about the size and shape of a pea, growing at the side of them. These are called Heberden's nodes, after the 16th century physician who first described them, and are often familial. They rarely lead to severe loss of function in the hand, but involvement of the carpo-metacarpal joint at the base of the thumb, which also occurs quite frequently, may be more incapacitating. The proximal interphalangeal (p.i.p.) and metacarpo-phalangeal (m.c.p.) joints may sometimes be involved by osteoarthrosis.

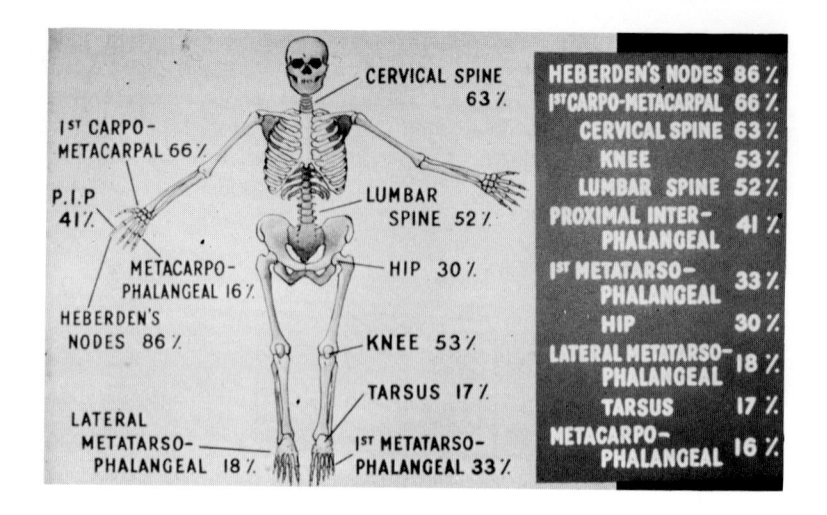

Fig. 4.4. The frequency of joints involved in patients with osteoarthrosis.

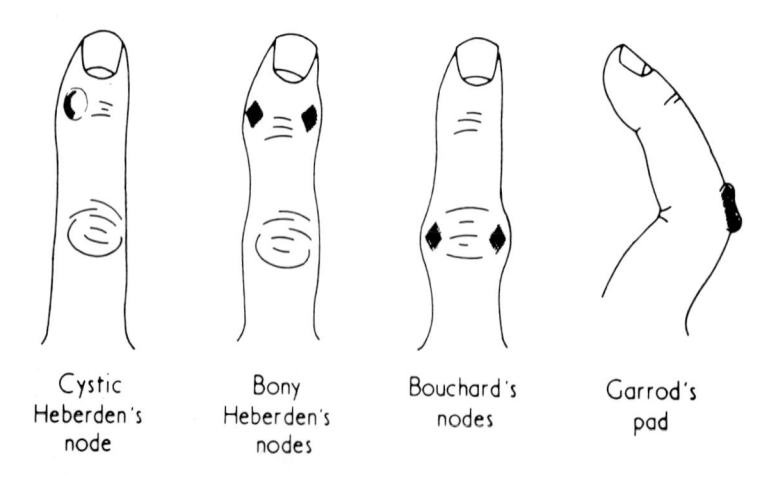

Fig. 4.5. Swellings of the finger in osteoarthrosis. 1) Heberden's nodes; 2) Bouchard's nodes; 3) Garrod's pads.

Secondary Osteoarthrosis

Any joint may be involved by secondary osteoarthrosis. Predisposing causes include previous fractures into the joint, which disturb the normal joint surface, or malalignment following a fracture leading to the forces through the joint acting in an unusual manner for which the joint is ill-constructed. Figure 4.6 shows osteoarthrosis in the right knee following an infected fracture in a man who was run over by a

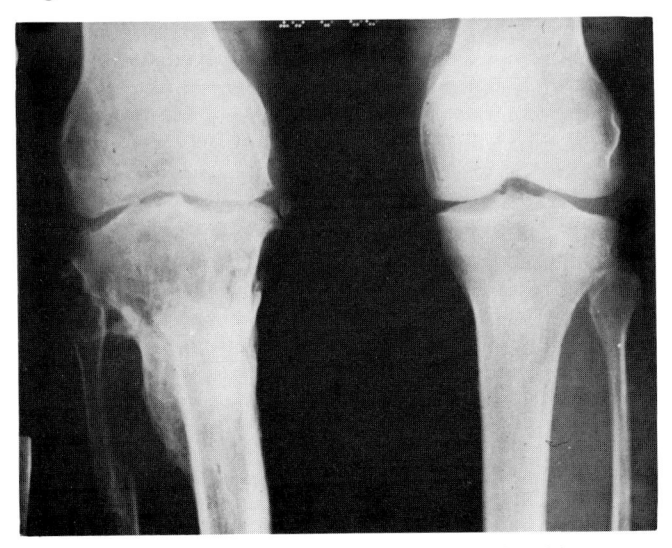

Fig. 4.6. Osteoarthrosis of knee following an infected knee.

steamwagon, contrasting with the normal appearance of the left knee. Osteoarthrosis in the hip may be associated with childhood disease such as congenital dislocation of the hip or Perthes's disease. It has recently been suggested that the modern tendency for young people with unfused epiphyses to undergo severe athletic training, particularly running for long distances on hard roads, may predispose them to developing osteoarthrosis in the hips in later life. Other causes of secondary osteoarthrosis include poliomyelitis, in which the normal leg is subjected to greater strain than the paralysed one because it is more capable of weight-bearing and therefore more used. In contrast, the paralysed limbs in poliomyelitis or hemiplegia are not usually affected by osteoarthrosis. Certain occupations lead to characteristic patterns of secondary osteoarthrosis. For example, colliers develop osteoarthrosis in their knees and elbows, and pneumatic drillers develop osteoarthrosis in their elbows. Some sporting activities also predispose to osteoarthrosis, such as that suffered by boxers or wicket keepers in their hands, and by judokas in their spines. Many patients suffering from osteoarthrosis of weightbearing joints, particularly the knee, are overweight and this should probably be thought of as osteoarthrosis secondary to their obesity.

Radiology

The appearances of osteoarthrosis on x-ray are those which would be expected from a knowledge of the pathology. The space between the bone ends on x-ray is the site of the articular cartilage. Because this allows x-rays through, it is termed radiolucent, and appears dark on the x-ray film. Bone, in contrast, stops x-rays to an extent which is proportional to its density, and therefore appears white on x-ray films. In osteoarthrosis the gap between the bone ends becomes narrower as the articular cartilage wears away. The increased bone density in the bone immediately beneath the cartilage, the subchondral bone, is represented by increased whiteness of the x-ray plate. The marginal osteophytes are seen as bony outgrowths, and bony, though not cartilaginous, loose bodies may be seen in the joint. As the disease advances the bone ends become increasingly deformed. Figures 4.7 and 4.8 show the radiological changes of osteoarthrosis of the hips and

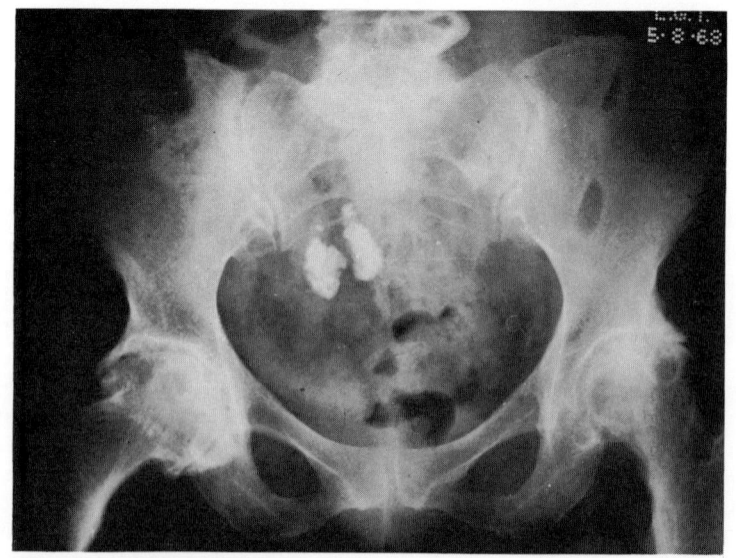

Fig. 4.7. Osteoarthrosis of hips, showing cysts in the bone, loss of joint space, sclerosis and osteophytes.

Osteoarthrosis

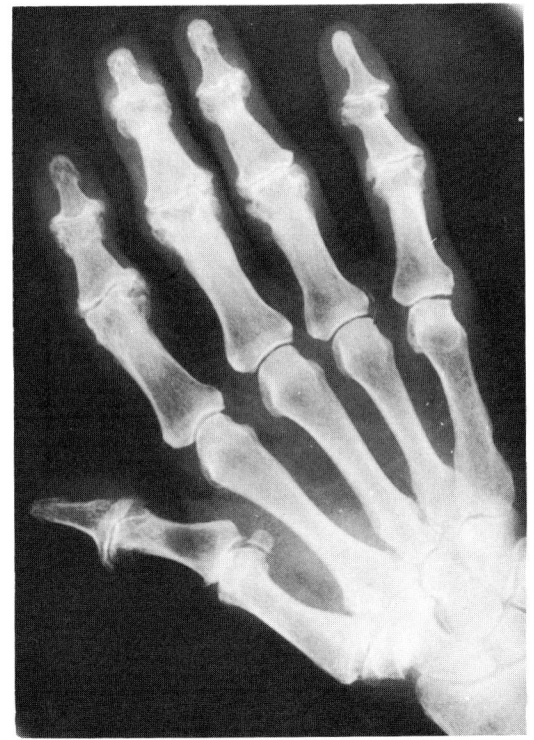

Fig. 4.8. Heberden's nodes, Bouchard's nodes of the proximal inter-phalangeal joint of the thumb and the first carpo-metacarpal joint.

hands. The diagnosis of osteoarthrosis is often made radiologically, as there are no characteristic laboratory abnormalities in this disease. Although there is a tendency for symptoms to increase as the radiological severity of the disease increases, it should be remembered that the presence of osteoarthrotic changes on x-ray does not of necessity mean that these are the cause of the patient's symptoms, as radiological osteoarthrosis may be asymptomatic (Fig. 4.9). The weightbearing joints are more likely to give symptoms when radiological changes are present than the joints of the arm.

Treatment

There are two important considerations in the treatment of osteoarthrosis. Firstly, in contrast to rheumatoid arthritis, this is a disease of joints alone rather than a generalised disease. Secondly, the prognosis in this condition is, in general, good, although some patients who might do badly are considered separately later. In general patients should avoid prolonged periods of immobilisation whether this is at home, at work or in hospital. This and other points regarding osteoarthrosis and its management are well illustrated in the booklet

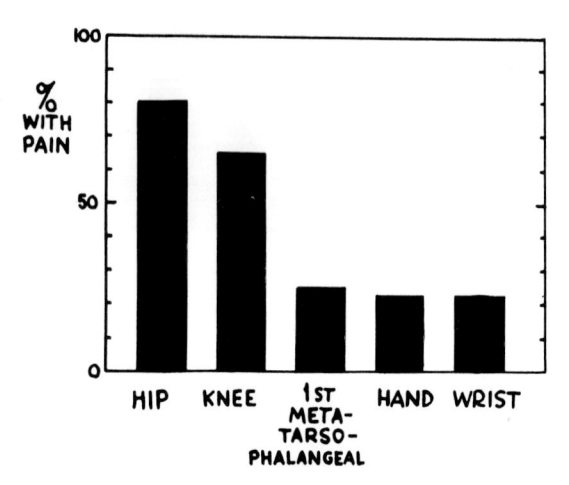

Fig. 4.9. Pain related to x-ray evidence of osteoarthrosis.

for patients with osteoarthrosis published by the Arthritis and Rheumatism Council. One exception to the stress on alternating periods of rest and exercise is that first carpo-metacarpal joints frequently do well after a period of immobilisation in plaster of Paris.

Symptomatic relief is afforded by the use of analgesics or analgesic/anti-inflammatory drugs. These are considered in detail in Chapter 21. The use of drugs which are pure analgesics is more common in osteoarthrosis than the other rheumatic diseases because of the small part played by the inflammatory process in the disease. In general, however, the analgesic/anti-inflammatory drugs of the aspirin type are used in treatment. Extra care must be taken in using phenylbutazone or its derivatives (the pyrazoles) in patients with osteoarthrosis. These are generally elderly people with a chronic disease, and prolonged use of these drugs in elderly patients is a known cause of aplastic anaemia. There is no place in the treatment of osteoarthrosis for the anti-inflammatory agents such as systemic corticosteroids, gold or antimalarials. The place of intra-articular injections of corticosteroids is very limited. They may be used occasionally in the treatment of an acute flare up of the disease, particularly in the first carpo-metacarpal joint, but injections during the non-inflammatory phase of the disease are not only no better than placebo injections but may cause damage to the joint. A more logical form of intra-articular therapy which has been suggested recently is the use of synthetic lubricants in osteoarthrotic joints. Unfortunately the first to be tried, silicone, was held to be effective on the basis of uncontrolled trials. In a controlled trial we undertook it was in fact less effective than normal saline. Research is continuing on more scientifically based synthetic lubricants.

Diet is not involved in the causation of osteoarthrosis, and its only place in treatment is weight reduction in the obese. Physiotherapy is often useful both in alleviating pain in the joints and, more particularly, in strengthening muscles and increasing the range of movement. Patients with osteoarthrosis of the hip may do especially well when treated in a hydrotherapy pool. The warmth of the water helps to relax muscle spasm and the buoyancy reduces the weight borne by the joint and enables freer movement. One important nursing point is that when a flexion deformity of the hip is present, the patient should be nursed prone for periods (e.g. an hour after meals).

Although the prognosis of osteoarthrosis in general is good, patients with osteoarthrosis of the hip may fare rather worse than the others. Disease in this joint tends to cause immobilisation, and as the disease advances these patients are particularly prone to difficulties at toilet and in sexual activities. Fortunately they are the group of patients for whom the most effective surgery is available.

Surgery

Surgical treatment is playing an increasing part in the management of osteoarthrosis. Initially the only widely used operation was osteotomy of the hip of the McMurray type, which sometimes produced relief of pain but did not, of course, significantly affect the range of movement. More recently interest has swung towards the use of total joint replacements (arthroplasties) for the hip joint. These usually comprise either a metal replacement for the femoral head articulating in a plastic acetabulum (the Charnley type prosthesis) or a metal femoral head articulating in a metal acetabulum (the McKee-Farrar or Ring type prosthesis). In general the results of implanting these prostheses, particularly the Charnley type, are excellent both in terms of pain relief and restoring mobility to the joint.

In contrast to the hip the most successful type of surgery currently practiced in the knee is osteotomy. This either takes the form of a tibial osteotomy or a double osteotomy in which both the femur and the tibia are cut. These appear to be an effective way of relieving pain, in about

60% of patients, although they do not increase the range of movement. The operation is particularly useful in a stable joint which shows marked deformity such as knock-knee. The results of total knee replacement are not yet sufficiently encouraging to make this as widely used an operation as hip replacement. There are many centres devising knee prostheses, and it is hoped that some more generally applicable models will soon be available. Surgery is discussed more fully in Chapter 22.

5
Infective Arthritis

Arthralgia and Myalgia in Infections
Arthritis as a Part of Infectious Diseases
  Enteric infections
  Brucellosis
  Reiter's disease
  Gonorrhoea
  Syphilis
  Whipple's disease
Joint Infections
  Brucella
  Tuberculosis
  Septic arthritis

Many people experience arthralgia (aching in the joints) or myalgia (aching in the muscles) during the course of infections. Less commonly the musculo-skeletal symptoms form a well-recognised part of an infectious disease, and rarely the joint itself may be the site of an infection.

Arthralgia and Myalgia in Infections

The aching limbs of the 'flu' syndrome, usually due to a virus infection though not always influenza virus, are well known. As the fever subsides, the aching in muscles and joints disappears, although the lethargy which follows an acute infection is often associated with a feeling of weakness in the muscles.

    Viral infections may, however, give rise to a marked synovitis which may mimic the early stages of rheumatoid arthritis. The best-known cause of this is rubella (German measles), where the arthritis, when present, is often the most distressing part of the illness, but other viral diseases, such as mumps, may give rise to a similar clinical picture. The diagnosis may be puzzling where the original illness was transient and trivial. In all cases the disease is self-limiting, the most valuable therapy being reassurance that no permanent arthritis will result, plus aspirin for symptomatic relief. Myalgic pains are most prominent in Bornholm disease. This condition, named after the Danish island from which the first epidemic was reported, is caused by infection with the Coxsackie virus. The pains, usually felt in the muscles of the chest wall, may be agonising and are accompanied by a constricting feeling during their exacerbation by respiration. This symptom-complex has been called 'devil's grip'. The pains may take several weeks to abate, and the feeling of weakness and malaise which follows may last for several months.

Arthritis as a Part of Infectious Diseases

A number of infections give rise to a 'reactive' synovitis in the joints. Although there may be evidence of blood-borne organisms during the acute phase of these diseases, the majority of cases of synovitis are not associated with the presence of infection in the joint. In some of these conditions, however, frank infection occurs.

Enteric infections

Infections such as salmonellal diarrhoea cause a synovitis in about 2.5% of cases. This usually occurs between 5 and 14 days after the initial infection, and may resemble rheumatoid arthritis. Occasionally the initial attack of diarrhoea may have been mild, and the diagnosis can only be made by careful history-taking or a knowledge of the presence of a local epidemic of diarrhoea. The arthritis is self-limiting, settling in days or, at most, weeks. The joints involved are shown in Fig. 5.1.

Brucellosis

Brucellosis (undulant fever) causes arthralgia in about one third of cases, especially during febrile periods. It may be contracted by drinking unpasteurised milk. Some patients go on to develop a more severe, chronic joint disease with x-ray evidence of joint damage.

Reiter's disease

This is a chronic polyarthritis which may affect the spine and is considered by some people as a 'variant' of ankylosing spondylitis. Certainly the advanced stage of Reiter's disease and ankylosing spondylitis may be identical. The classical triad of symptoms of Reiter's disease comprises urethritis, conjunctivitis, and arthritis, though

Infective Arthritis

occasionally one of these may be absent. The disease follows one of two conditions, either dysentery (the post-dysenteric form) or sexually-transmitted urethritis (the post-sexual form). Although the largest series of reported cases all followed dysentery, the post-sexual form of the disease is the more common in the United Kingdom. Indeed it is the greatest hazard to which the promiscuous male is subject in Britain. The arthritis may vary from a mild polyarthritis, which subsides spontaneously, to a severe and crippling disease.

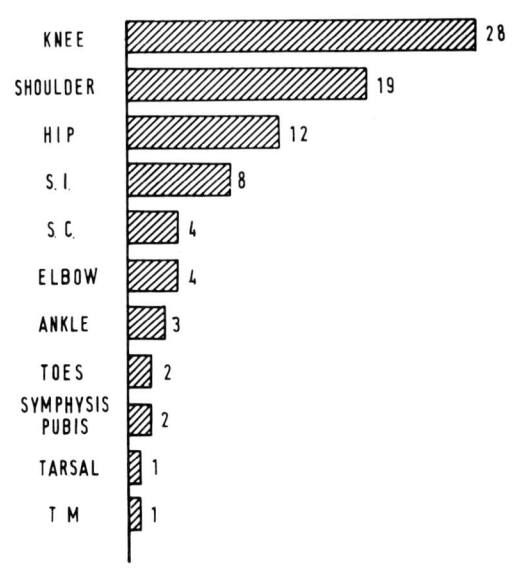

Joint	Number
KNEE	28
SHOULDER	19
HIP	12
S.I.	8
S.C.	4
ELBOW	4
ANKLE	3
TOES	2
SYMPHYSIS PUBIS	2
TARSAL	1
TM	1

Fig. 5.1. Salmonella arthritis—joints affected in 54 patients.

The large weightbearing joints, especially the knees, are the most commonly involved (Fig. 5.2). The ankles, elbows, and wrists may also be affected. Reiter's disease is the cause of some of the largest joint effusions seen in rheumatological practice, and aspiration of tense effusions often provides considerable relief to the patient. Where sacro-iliac and spinal involvement occur, the treatment of this aspect of the disease is the same as that of ankylosing spondylitis. A number of other signs may occur during the course of Reiter's disease. These include oral and genital ulceration, a characteristic rash called keratoderma blenorrhagica (Fig. 5.3) on the palms and soles, and pain in the heels which is often accompanied by the presence of plantar spurs on x-ray (Fig. 5.4).

Gonorrhoea

Other venereal infections may also be associated with arthritis. Gonorrhoea may be accompanied by an arthritis, often involving one joint only, or by tenosynovitis. Patients who have skin lesions as a part of their gonococcal infection are particularly liable to develop joint disease. The gonococcus is a difficult organism to culture, but some joint fluid aspirates have grown gonococci and it is possible that the majority of these cases are, in fact, infective.

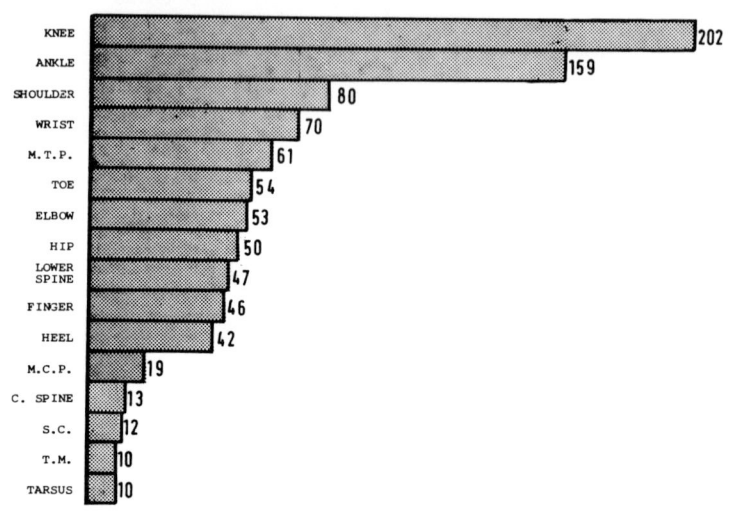

Joint	Count
KNEE	202
ANKLE	159
SHOULDER	80
WRIST	70
M.T.P.	61
TOE	54
ELBOW	53
HIP	50
LOWER SPINE	47
FINGER	46
HEEL	42
M.C.P.	19
C. SPINE	13
S.C.	12
T.M.	10
TARSUS	10

Fig. 5.2. Reiter's disease—joints affected in course of disease.

Gonococcal arthritis and tenosynovitis are diagnosed more often in the southern states of the USA than in Britain. Although some recent studies suggest that this condition is underdiagnosed in this country, there is probably a true difference in incidence of the disease. It should, however, be remembered as a possible cause of an unexplained arthritis.

Syphilis

The incidence of syphilis is declining and treatment has improved in recent years. The joint manifestations of syphilis are, therefore, increasingly uncommon, and are now usually found in old cases. With the virtual disappearance of congenital syphilis, the bilateral knee effusions (Clutton's joints) found in this condition have become almost extinct, although they still appear in lists of differential diagnoses of Still's disease. Secondary syphilis may be accompanied by arthralgia during the febrile stage. Synovitis, especially of the knees, may also occur during the course of secondary syphilis. It is self-limiting, but may persist for up to a year. Charcot joints are still seen in patients with tertiary syphilis. In this condition there is gross destruction, usually of

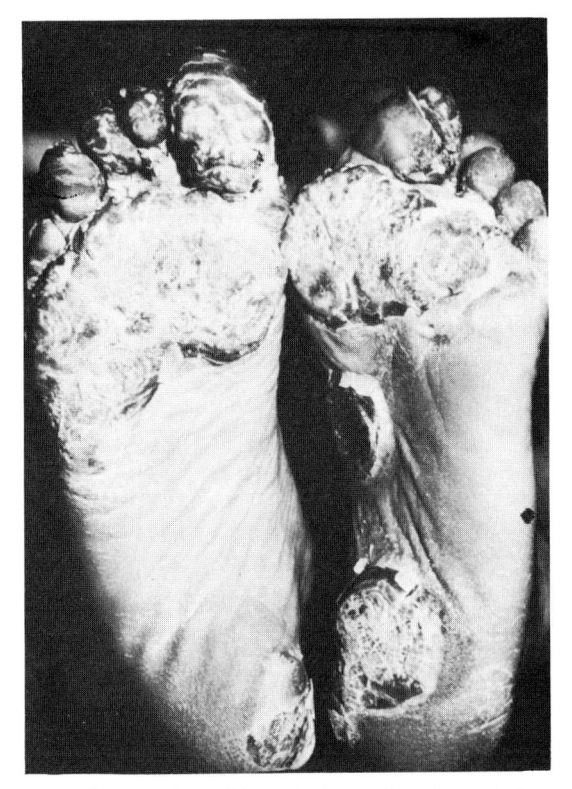

Fig. 5.3. Keratoderma blenorrhagica on the soles of the feet of a patient with Reiter's disease.

one joint. This occurs where there is involvement of the nervous system as part of the syphilitic process, producing tabes dorsalis. The loss of sensation from the joint allows it to become damaged by unrealised trauma. Although these joints are usually painless, especially late in the disease, they may be markedly painful in some patients.

Whipple's disease

This is a rare condition in which an intestinal disease that appears to be due to an infection is associated in most cases with a polyarthritis. The importance of the arthritis is that in many cases it precedes the development of intestinal symptoms, occasionally by several years. The joints affected are those of the lower limb rather than the small upper-limb joints. X-rays show no damage to these joints, but sacroiliitis may occasionally be seen.

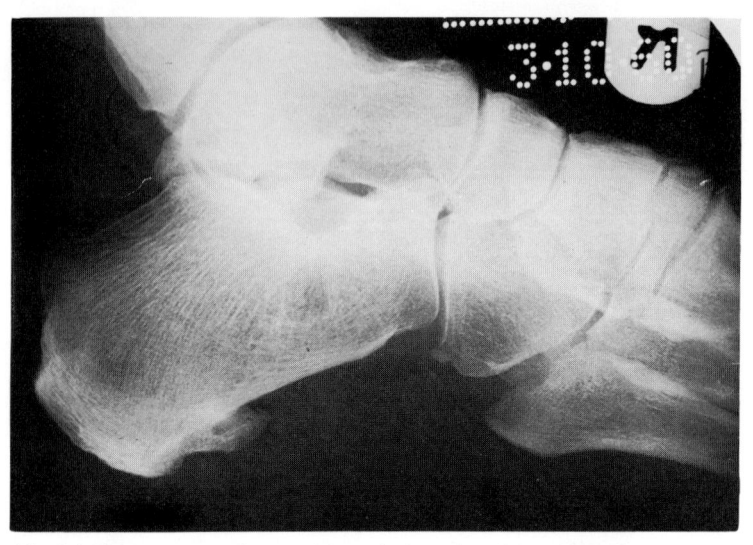

Fig. 5.4. Plantar spur on the os calcis at the insertion of the plantar fascia in a bus driver with Reiter's syndrome.

Joint Infections

Infection within a joint is a dangerous condition. It may destroy the joint and occasionally threaten the life of the patient. The enteric diseases mentioned earlier may, on rare occasions, cause direct infection of a joint. In contrast with the more transient synovitis already described, direct infection is usually localised to one joint, where there are signs of severe inflammation with pain, redness, and swelling of a joint that is noticeably warm to the touch. The organisms in direct infection may reach the joint by a wound from the outside, from adjacent infected bone or other tissue, or by bacteria circulating in the bloodstream. The diagnosis is confirmed by culture of the offending organism from the joint aspirate.

Treatment comprises rest of the infected joint and administration of systemic antibiotics. It is now known that antibiotics penetrate into the joint cavity when given by their usual oral or intramuscular routes. It is, therefore, not necessary to inject antibiotics directly into the joints, although aspiration of thick pus, either with a wide-bore needle or by surgery, may be needed.

For diagnostic purposes aspiration of the joints is essential, and in this way the organism can be isolated and the sensitivity to antibiotics determined.

Brucella

This may also cause an infective arthritis, and this occasionally involves the sacro-iliac joints or the spine. It may cause osteomyelitis in adjacent bones, which will require the usual surgical treatment.

Tuberculosis

Tuberculosis may act in a similar way, producing an infective arthritis either in peripheral joints or the spine. Although the incidence of tuberculosis has declined considerably since the introduction of tuberculin testing of cattle, BCG vaccination in humans, and effective antituberculous medication, this disease still affects a large number of people in Britain each year. The immigrant population is particularly liable. The arthritis may occur during the course of a known tuberculous infection and is treated with rest and appropriate antibiotics. Patients, however, present themselves with tuberculous infection in their joints. As with tuberculosis elsewhere, the onset may be slow and silent. This especially applies in children, where the hip, which is not easily inspected, is the joint most commonly involved. By the time the child presents himself, often with a painless limp, severe joint destruction may have taken place. The hip is also the most commonly affected joint in the adult, although the knee and other peripheral joints may also be affected. Chemotherapy may be sufficient to prevent serious joint destruction, provided it is started early enough in the course of the disease. If there is existing joint damage, however, surgery may be necessary.

Tuberculous infection may also involve the spine (Pott's disease). The focus of infection appears to be within the vertebral body, spreading from there into the disc. The infected material may press backwards into the spinal canal, resulting in neurological signs or even paraplegia. A so-called 'cold abscess' may track down the psoas sheath and point in the groin. (It is called 'cold' because it may not have many of the signs of associated inflammation, e.g., it may not be warm or red.) Collapse of the destroyed vertebrae gives rise to the characteristic gibbus deformity of the back. In the treatment of tuberculosis of the spine, in which prolonged immobilisation may be necessary, some of the worst problems of prolonged bed rest have been found. In particular, patients so immobilised are very liable to develop renal calculi, and for this reason many devices to give movement to the bedfast patient, such as rocking beds, have been devised in order to try and minimise such complications. This is one of the reasons why modern treatment aims at keeping such patients in bed for as short a period as possible, supporting the spine surgically if necessary, to allow mobilisation.

Septic arthritis

This occurs when a joint is infected with a pyogenic organism. The possibility that some or many cases of gonococcal arthritis may in fact be due to direct infection has already been discussed. Meningococci also give rise to an arthritis which usually occurs in association with meningococcal meningitis. As with most people with meningitis or septicaemia there is frequently arthralgia and myalgia in the early course of the disease, but occasionally a single joint shows signs of local infection and meningococci may be isolated from it.

The majority of cases of septic arthritis arise in patients who are in some way predisposed to infection. These include the very young, particularly premature babies, and the very old. Patients suffering from debilitating diseases and from diabetes mellitus may also develop septic joints. Patients with rheumatoid arthritis, however, form the group in whom the majority of cases of septic arthritis arise. It is important to be aware of the possibility of this complication of rheumatoid arthritis, as the diagnosis may be difficult. Although most cases affect one joint, the knee being the most common, many are mis-diagnosed as a flare-up of the rheumatoid disease.

The signs of an infected joint—pain, redness, swelling, warmth, and loss of function—may occur in a non-infected rheumatoid joint, thus complicating the diagnosis. The diagnosis is made by aspirating the joint and growing the infecting organism from it. The source of the sepsis may be quite trivial, such as a boil or an infected lesion between the toes. Some patients have an ulcerated nodule or chest infection, while others show no obvious point of entry. It seems likely that organisms escape from such sites into the bloodstream in most people, but the lush rheumatoid synovium provides a site where they can reproduce without being taken up by scavenging white cells. Other joints apart from the knee may be involved. In a series of patients, the knee was infected in five, but the hip, shoulder, elbow, wrist, sternoclavicular joint, and ankle were involved in others. The sternoclavicular joint appears to be particularly liable to infection with staphylococci, which are the commonest of the infecting organisms. Although *staphylococci, streptococci, pneumococci,* and *E. coli* are the commonest infecting organisms, septic arthritis is showing the same trend as other forms of focal infection, in that the types of organisms which may cause it appear to be increasing. Thus rarer Gram-negative organisms, yeasts, and fungi may be involved in joint infections, possibly reflecting the change brought about by widespread use of antibiotics in the community. In our series, men had infected joints four times more commonly than women, the average age was 52 years, nodules were present in half, and the arthritis was moderate or severe in extent, having been present for an average of 14 years.

Treatment of septic arthritis is by identification of the organism and a course of the appropriate antibiotic. The joint should be rested during the acute phase, although passive movements should be undertaken daily. Repeated joint aspiration and local instillation of antibiotics is no longer considered necessary, as most antibiotics penetrate adequately into the synovial fluid.

Two aspects of the treatment of rheumatoid arthritis help to make these patients particularly liable to joint infections. The first is the use of intra-articular therapy. The technique for this will be described in Chapter 20, p. 200, but it is important that an aseptic technique is used, as organisms may otherwise be introduced into the joint.

The systemic use of corticosteroids also predisposes to joint infections as well as infections elsewhere, although in our series two-thirds of the patients were not on steroids at the time of infection. An additional danger is that the use of corticosteroids may minimise the local signs of inflammation. The less widely used cytotoxic drugs also interfere with the body's capacity to deal with invading organisms and therefore predispose to infective arthritis. These drugs are relatively more widely used in the treatment of leukaemia and in patients undergoing renal transplantation. Both these groups of patients are also susceptible to infective arthritis.

6
Ankylosing Spondylitis

Pathology
Prevalence
Clinical Features
Physical Signs
Prognosis
Complications
Blood Tests
X-ray Changes
Treatment

Although ankylosing spondylitis is uncommon it is important. Much can be done to benefit the sufferer and wrong treatment can do great harm. The disease is sometimes popularly known as 'poker pack' because of the rigidity it may produce in the spine. It is an inflammatory arthritis of the spine, involving the sacro-iliac joints (at the junction of the spine and pelvis) and less commonly the peripheral joints. The disease affects predominantly young men in their twenties and is usually self-limiting. Its cause is unknown.

Pathology

The main changes occur in the spine. The sacro-iliac joints are involved and then other spinal structures such as the annulus fibrosus, which forms the outer surrounding of the intervertebral disc, become calcified. The joints between the vertebrae of the back, apophyseal joints, become inflamed and then eroded. These changes tend to spread up the spine involving first the lumbar region, then the dorsal region, and finally the cervical spine. This order of involvement may not always occur however. When peripheral joints are involved, inflammation of the synovium produces a synovitis and there may be an excess of fluid exuded into the joint cavity. The inflammation is similar to that of rheumatoid arthritis, although there tends to be more fibrosis. Where ligaments attach to bone there is often inflammation as well, producing a reaction that leads on to bone changes or calcification.

Prevalence

In the general population it affects about one in 200 men and one in 2,000 women. Some groups of people seem particularly prone to it and a group of Red Indians in British Columbia are more frequently affected. There is also an hereditary element and relatives of patients with ankylosing spondylitis are more likely to show the disease. There are a number of other conditions with which it is associated, such as psoriasis, ulcerative colitis, Crohn's disease and Reiter's syndrome. In the case of Reiter's syndrome it has been suggested that the infection (whether acquired venereally or arising from the bowel following dysentery) has a fairly direct relationship. In other conditions, however, the spondylitis may precede the skin or bowel condition. It is thought that there are genetic factors which predispose to these various diseases and there is an overlap of the predisposing genetic factors— what is known as an overlap of the gene pool. The disease affects men more frequently than women in a clinic population as well as in the general population. Our figures showed that 79% were men and 21% women. It has been suggested that the women get the disease less severely and this is the reason why they present less frequently to the clinic.

Clinical Features

The disease is particularly seen in young men (Fig. 6.1). Most patients begin with pain in the lower part of their back accompanied by stiffness

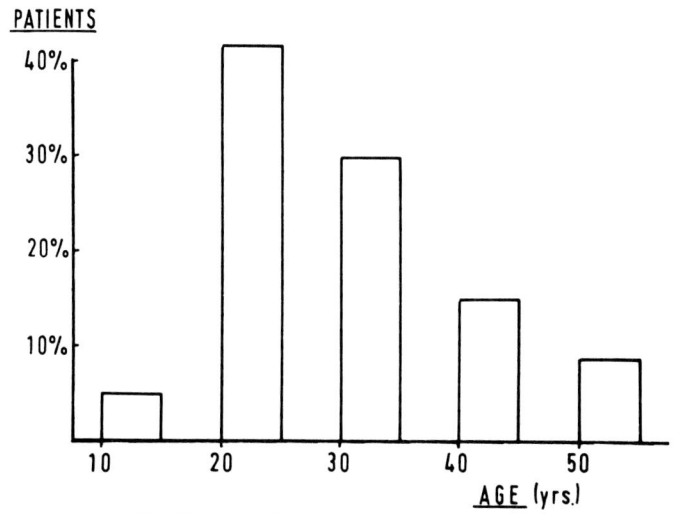

Fig. 6.1. Age of onset of ankylosing spondylitis.

which is worst in the early morning. In contrast to a 'slipped disc', in which rest in bed alleviates symptoms, the pain and stiffness are aggravated in ankylosing spondylitis by rest. Occasionally the presenting symptom may be a synovitis of the knee, or an iritis (Fig. 6.2). The disease usually comes on gradually and may mimic other diseases,

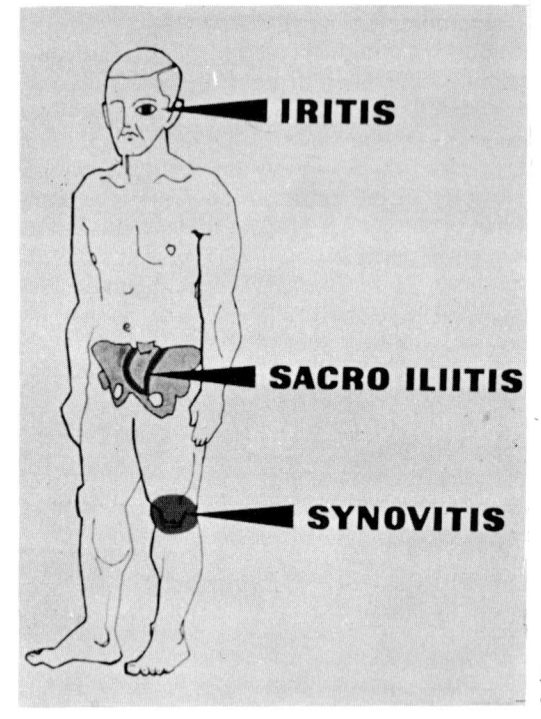

Fig. 6.2. Presenting features of ankylosing spondylitis.

because of the radiation of the pain (Fig. 6.3). In 10% of patients the pain radiates down the back of the legs and a slipped disc may be misdiagnosed. On other occasions it may radiate around the loin and kidney disease be suspected. Because of involvement of the costo-vertebral joints (where the ribs join the spine) pain may radiate around the chest. There is also rigidity of chest movement so that chest expansion is limited. Because of this, breathing is largely diaphragmatic and there may be ballooning of the abdomen on breathing. There may be constitutional symptoms, such as loss of appetite and loss of weight, and occasionally a raised temperature.

Ankylosing Spondylitis

Physical Signs

There may be few physical signs in the early stage of ankylosing spondylitis. We have a number of patients with a typical history of back pain and stiffness, classical x-ray changes, but little in the way of abnormal posture or mobility. The sacro-iliac joints may be tender. Later the lumbar lordosis (the normal curve in the lower part of the back) is lost and movement of the lumbar spine becomes limited in all

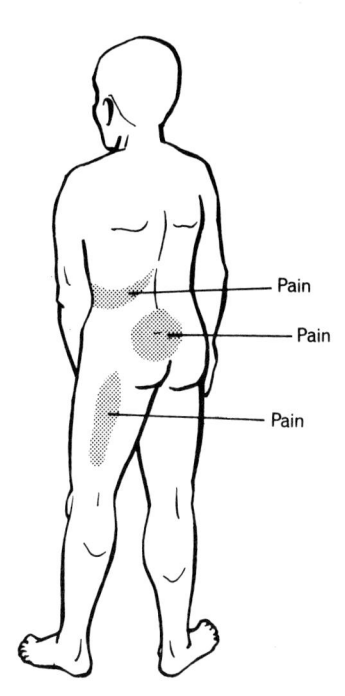

Fig. 6.3. Radiation of pain in ankylosing spondylitis.

directions. When the back becomes completely rigid it is known as a 'poker back'. The limitation of movement usually begins in the lumbar region and is accompanied by spasm in the muscles alongside the spine (paravertebral muscle spasm). The limitation of movement may extend up the spine to include the neck. As the disease advances the patients may develop a stoop (Fig. 6.4). Because of the involvement of the costo-vertebral joints, chest expansion becomes limited.

When peripheral joints are involved it is usually larger joints such as hips and shoulders that are affected. Other joints such as the knees, ankles, elbows and wrists may also be involved, and less commonly, the small joints of the hands and feet. The hip disease is particularly important as it may interfere with walking and if flexion contractures develop posture is affected. Flexion contractures at the hip necessitate flexion at the knee to maintain an erect posture and this profile with bent hips and knees in spondylitics has been described as resembling a letter Z. In advanced disease, therefore, the patient may have a

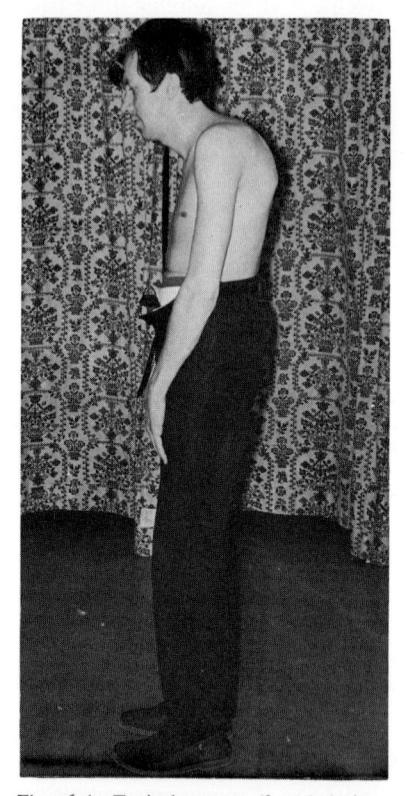

Fig. 6.4. Typical stoop of ankylosing spondylitis.

'hang-dog' appearance and a wide based stance. There is forward craning of the neck, high dorsal kyphosis, rounding of the shoulders, straight or even convex lumbar spine, wasted buttocks, flattening of the chest and ballooning of the abdomen. The visual field may be so restricted that prismatic spectacles have to be provided to permit forward vision.

Prognosis

The modern treatment of ankylosing spondylitis has revolutionised the outlook. Rarely is the severe disease described above seen. Indeed, 85% of these patients never lose a day from work. In only about 5% of patients does the disease take an unfavourable course from the onset, and in these subjects permanent invalidism due to widespread ankylosis occurs within a few years. Often the patients have so little trouble that the symptoms pass unnoticed until drawn to their attention. It has been shown in a group of hospital patients that two-thirds or more were able to support themselves and their families after twenty years of symptoms.

Complications

It used to be thought that pulmonary tuberculosis was more common and chest infections more frequent in these patients, but that does not seem to be so. They may however have a dislocation of the neck vertebrae, or subluxation between the atlas and axis vertebrae. This can give paraplegia. Iritis occurs in 10-20% and on rare occasions produces blindness. Amyloidosis (the deposition of an abnormal protein in various tissues) sometimes occurs. The aortic valve is involved in about 4% of patients. Some other complications are related to therapy.

Blood Tests

There is often a mild degree of anaemia, and in the majority of cases the erythrocyte sedimentation rate (ESR) is raised. Occasionally there is an increased white cell count (leucocytosis). Tests for rheumatoid factor are negative, and this helps to distinguish the disease from rheumatoid arthritis, with which in the USA it was confused for a number of years, being termed 'rheumatoid spondylitis' on that side of the Atlantic. There has been much interest in the discovery over the last two or three years that a special tissue antigen (histocompatibility antigen), denoted HLA-B27, is positive in 90% of these patients. It indicates an hereditary predisposition to the disease.

X-ray Changes

The sacro-iliac joints are involved with sclerosis and erosion (Fig. 6.5) and at a later stage ankylosis (Fig. 6.6). Later the spine becomes involved with calcification of the outer portion of the annulus fibrosus of the intervertebral disc (Fig. 6.7). The apophyseal joints of the back of

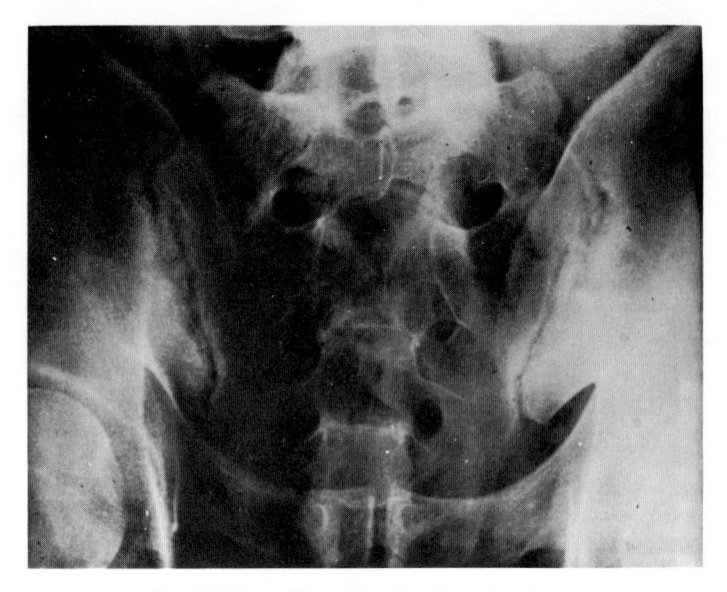

Fig. 6.5. Sacro-iliitis with sclerosis and erosion.

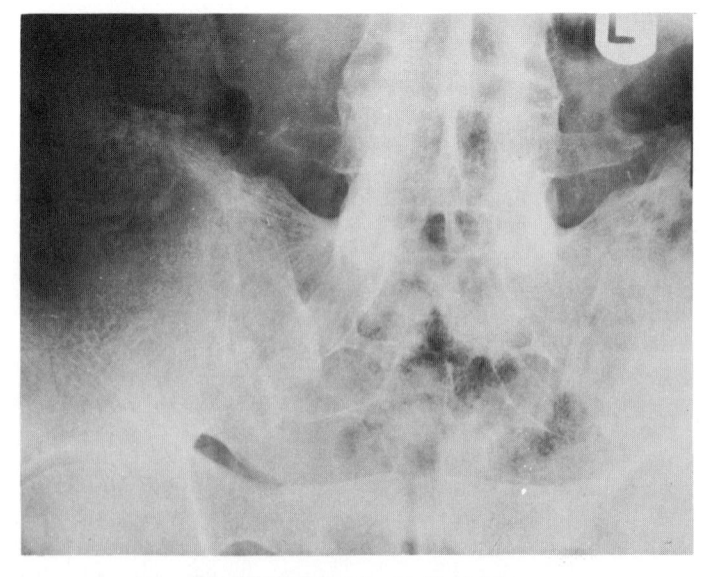

Fig. 6.6. Ankylosed sacro-iliac joints.

Ankylosing Spondylitis

the vertebrae are also involved. The calcification gives rise to the typical 'bamboo spine'. Although peripheral joints are involved clinically they may not show very marked changes radiographically.

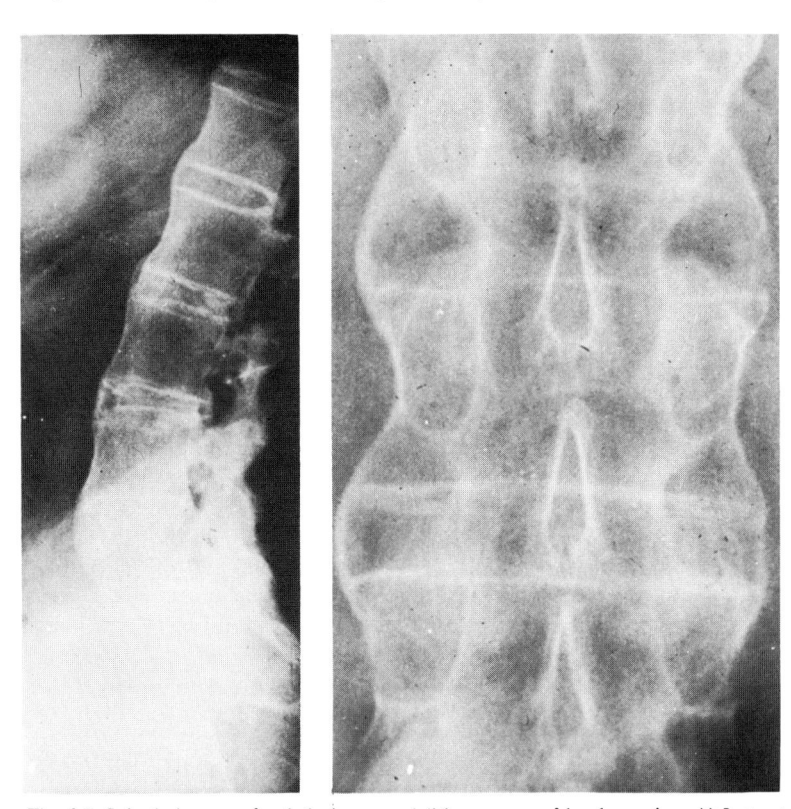

Fig. 6.7. Spinal changes of ankylosing spondylitis on x-ray of lumbar spine. A) Lateral view. B) Posterior view.

Treatment

This is the one rheumatic disease above all others where mobilisation is vital. Years ago these patients were encased in plaster casts to prevent deformity. Inexorably they bent and cracked the cast, leaving permanent flexion deformities of the spine. We now know that this is quite the wrong way to treat these patients. They must be taught a regime of exercises, with maintenance of posture and increase of chest expansion. They should be encouraged to do these regularly at home. Our policy is to give all patients with ankylosing spondylitis a course of instruction in the Physiotherapy Department for this purpose. The patient should lie in a good position in bed and fracture boards under the mattress are often helpful. Hydrotherapy in the deep pool is beneficial and swimming is an exercise that should be encouraged since it is not weight bearing. A very good booklet for patients, published by the Arthritis and Rheumatism Council, is often given by doctors; it explains the nature of the disease and gives points about general management.

Analgesics are prescribed during the active phase and typical drugs used are soluble aspirin, phenylbutazone, indomethacin and naproxen Corticosteroids are not commonly used, but may be necessary if the disease progresses inexorably or if the eyes are threatened by severe iritis.

Radiotherapy was commonly employed at one time, but since it has been appreciated that there is an increased risk of leukaemia in patients so treated it is less frequently advocated. It should be appreciated that, although the risk of leukaemia is increased ten-fold, the incidence is still only 0.15% of patients treated. This is a mortality rate lower than one may expect with corticosteroid treatment. It is important therefore to see this problem in perspective. Observations following the atomic bomb explosion at Hiroshima, as well as those on spondylitic patients treated with radiotherapy, showed that the higher the dose of radiation the more likely was the person to develop leukaemia. Many doctors would be prepared, therefore, to give a single course of radiotherapy in patients who are not responding to treatment.

Surgery is occasionally employed. The risks are high for endeavours to straighten the spine, and this is only occasionally attempted. Where the hips are involved a Charnley arthroplasty to replace these has proved very successful for some of our patients.

7
Degenerative Disease of the Spine

Anatomy
Pathology
Clinical Features
Investigations
Treatment
 Rest and traction
 Physiotherapy
 Drug therapy
 Surgery

Degenerative disease in the spine is common. National insurance figures for 1970/71 showed 13.7 million days lost from work due to back pain, and surveys suggest that this is probably an underestimate. In heavy manual workers one study found that 51% of sickness absence in the previous year had been due to back pain, totalling 225 weeks absence per 1000 men per year. The whole of the vertebral column may be involved, but most symptoms arise from the cervical and lumbar regions.

Two types of disease occur. True osteoarthrosis occurs in the spinal apophyseal joints. Degenerative disease in relation to the intervertebral discs is more correctly called spondylosis, but the changes and their effects are so similar that the two conditions are usually considered together.

Anatomy

In order to understand spinal disease, the anatomy of the vertebral column must be studied (Fig. 7.1). The spinal column consists of 33 vertebrae. Seven are cervical, 12 thoracic or dorsal (the names are used interchangeably), 5 lumbar, 5 sacral and 4 coccygeal. The sacral and coccygeal vertebrae normally fuse during development to form a solid block of bone. Quite frequently abnormalities of development occur in the low back. Although spina bifida is usually easily recognised, spina bifida occulta, in which there is a minor defect in formation of the vertebral arch, is often an incidental finding on x-ray. A tuft of hair at the base of the spine may be seen as an outer marker of this condition. The process of fusion of the sacrum should finish at the L.5/S.1 junction. This process may go wrong in two ways. If fusion stops short of the first sacral vertebra this is said to be lumbarised, that is, it is a

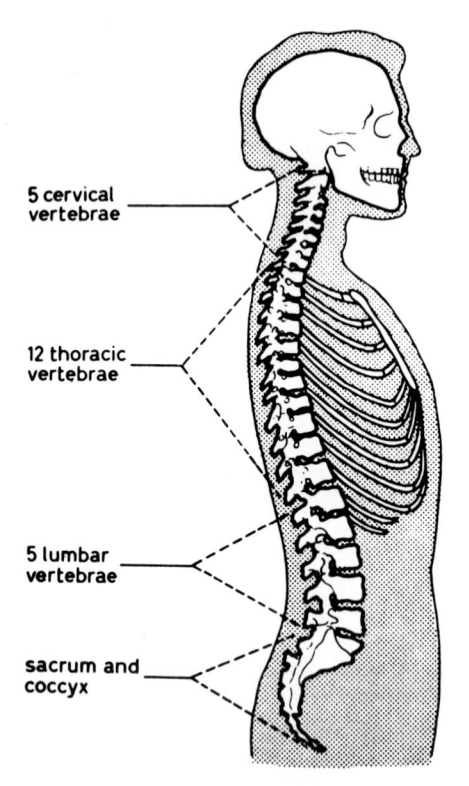

Fig. 7.1. The vertebral column.

separate vertebra apart from the sacral block. This may occur on one side of the spine only—hemi-lumbarisation. Alternatively the process of fusion may proceed to involve the fifth lumbar vertebra, which is then incorporated into the bony block. This is sacralisation of L.5 (Fig. 7.2) or, if only half the vertebra is involved, hemi-sacralisation. These minor abnormalities are usually held to be clinically insignificant, but hemi-sacralisation or lumbarisation may cause abnormal strains in the lower spine producing osteoarthrosis.

Degenerative Disease of the Spine

The vertebral column has three curves, one primary and two secondary. The primary curve is flexion of the whole spine, the posture of the fetus. The process of raising the head extends the neck and produces the first secondary curve, the cervical lordosis. The second secondary curve, the lumbar lordosis, appears with standing. Alteration of the spinal curves is frequently seen in patients with spinal pain. The

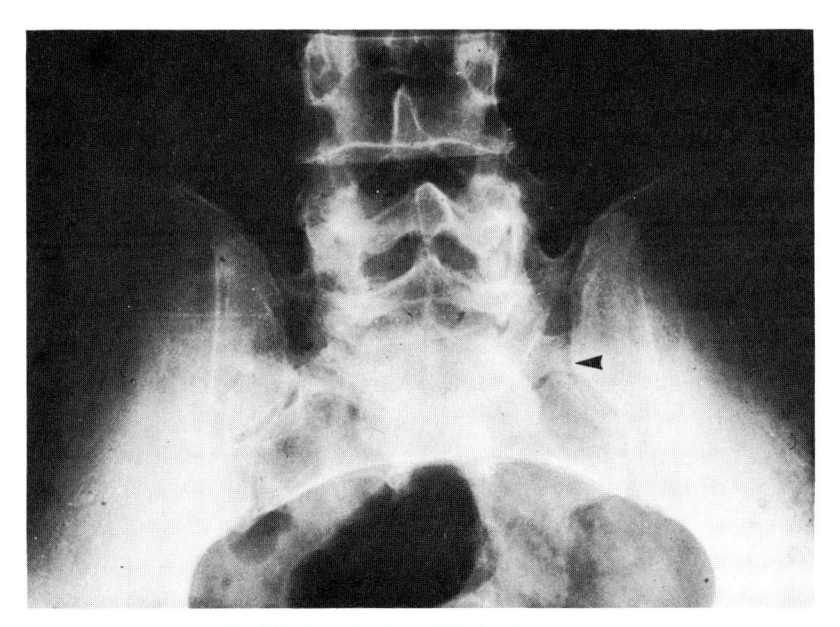

Fig. 7.2. Sacralization of 5th lumbar vertebra.

primary curve is often exaggerated to a dorsal kyphosis either by virtue of faulty posture or spinal disease. This has the consequence of exaggerating the cervical lordosis in order to allow the patient to look ahead. In such patients the change in posture exaggerates the normal prominence of the seventh cervical vertebra, the vertebra prominens. This is often considered by patients to be a pathological lump and identified as the source of their complaints.

The cervical lordosis may be straightened or reversed in patients with neck pain giving them an abject, hang-dog look. The rhythm of cervical movement is often altered due to splintage of the lowest three vertebrae because of spasm in the trapezius muscle. The lumbar lordosis may be exaggerated or reduced in patients with back pain. It is often difficult to decide whether these alterations in posture are the cause or effect of the pain.

The normal spinal curves are all antero-posterior. Lateral curvature is called scoliosis and is always abnormal. It may be due to a primary structural abnormality such as failure of rib development or secondary to muscle imbalance due either to unilateral weakness or spasm. In acute disc prolapse a sciatic scoliosis is produced in an attempt to relieve the pressure on the affected nerve root.

Although there are differences in the detailed anatomy of vertebra at different levels, their basic structure is the same throughout. The most anterior part is the vertebral body. This is the load bearing area of the vertebra and is separated from the vertebrae above and below by an intervertebral disc. Two arches curve backwards from the sides of the body and join posteriorly to form the spinous process. The gap formed by the two arches and the body contains the spinal cord. The apophyseal joints articulate between vertical extensions of the arch and articular facets on the spinous process of the vertebra above (Fig. 7.3).

The intervertebral disc provides mobility and cushioning to the spine. The outer annulus fibrosus is a strong meshwork of collagen fibres. The central nucleus pulposus is soft and gelatinous. This flattens under pressure and bulges outwards (Fig. 7.4). In pathological circumstances it may protrude through the annulus. Lying on a board may restore the situation.

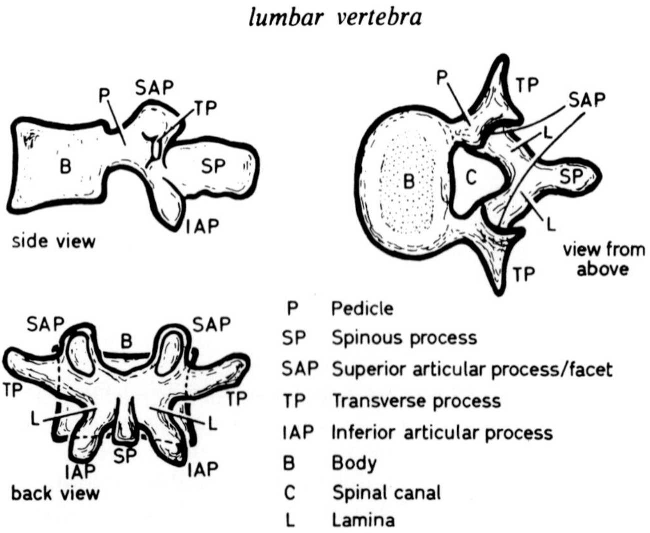

lumbar vertebra

P   Pedicle
SP Spinous process
SAP Superior articular process/facet
TP Transverse process
IAP Inferior articular process
B   Body
C   Spinal canal
L   Lamina

Fig. 7.3. Anatomy of vertebra.

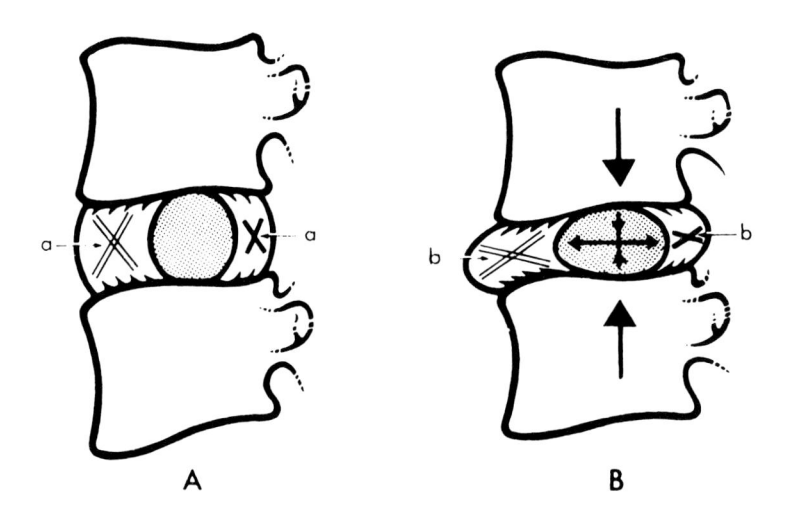

Fig. 7.4. Result of pressure on an invertebral disc.

Pathology

Various causes of backache occur at different ages generally and these are summarised in Table 7.1. In terms of frequency of presentation at our Back Pain Clinic the diagnoses are shown in Table 7.2. Of 8,541 patients admitted over a 5-year period to the Royal Bath Hospital, Harrogate, the diagnoses of spinal pain are shown in Table 7.3.

Where osteoarthrosis occurs, the pathological changes are similar to those seen elsewhere. Disc degeneration may result in protrusion of the nucleus through the annulus in any direction. Postero-lateral protrusion produces pressure on the nerve roots and posterior protrusions may press on the cord or cauda equina (Fig. 7.5). Where longstanding disc degeneration has occurred, narrowing of the disc occurs and changes similar to those of osteoarthrosis, appear in the vertebral bodies, with osteophyte formation which may be very large (Fig. 7.6). These osteophytes are bony outgrowths from the margin of the vertebral body. In our area disc prolapse was found at laminectomy at L.5/S.1 in 51%, L.4/5 in 43% and L.3/4 in 6.6%.

Minor congenital abnormalities of the back may predispose to backache. Back pain was found more frequently in 1,000 patients with sacralisation of a lumbar vertebra on one side that it was in 1,000 control subjects.

Backache Age of Onset/Diagnosis	
2—15 yr	Postural Osteochondritis
15—30	Spondylitis Prolapsed disc
30—50	Prolapsed disc Ochronosis
50+	Spondylosis Neoplasms Osteoporosis Paget's disease

Table 7.1 Causes of backache related to age.

Low Back Pain Diagnosis		
	Male	Female
Disc Disease	62	35
Trauma	23	18
Congenital Anomaly	28	17

Table 7.2 Diagnoses in patients with low back pain attending the Back Pain Clinic at Leeds.

Spinal Pain—RBH Registrations 5 yr Period	
Total Patients	8,541
Cervical	460
Dorsal	20
Low Back	481
Multiple	157
Ankylosing Spondylitis	84

Table 7.3 Diagnoses of spinal pain in 8,541 patients admitted to the Royal Bath Hospital, Harrogate. Where an anatomical site is listed, those patients had disc degeneration and/or osteoarthrosis.

Clinical Features

The clinical picture of degenerative spinal disease comprises a combination of local and referred pain. In our series the pain began suddenly in half the men and one third of the women. A history of injury was obtained in 60% of the men and 26% of the women. Unaccustomed activity, such as digging the garden, had preceded the episode in 16% of the patients.

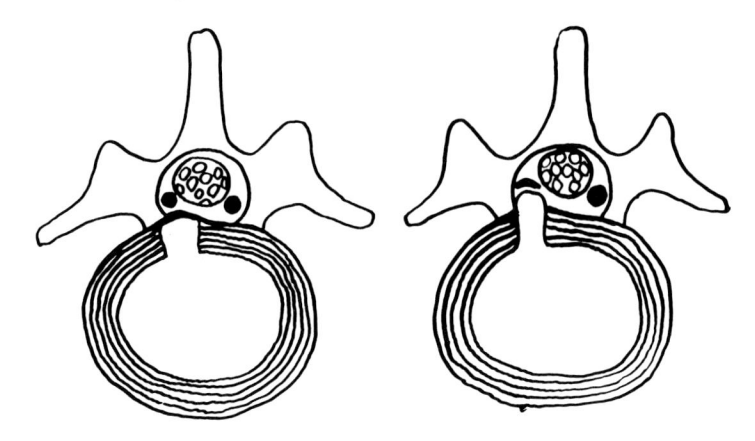

Fig. 7.5. Disc protrusion ('slipped disc').

In acute postero-lateral disc prolapse low back pain, often of sudden and dramatic onset, may be accompanied by radiation of pain to the appropriate segment of the lower limb, for example through the sciatic distribution where L.4/5 protrudes. The age distribution of those with and without sciatica differs and each sex has its own pattern (Fig. 7.7). In some patients, paraesthesiae rather than pain are felt in the leg, and back pain is occasionally minimal or absent. Examination reveals a rigid lumbar spine segment, often with a sciatic scoliosis which may be more prominent on attempted flexion. Straight leg raising on the affected side may be reduced and a neurological abnormality appropriate to the level of the lesion will be found. By straight leg raising pain may be produced; with a posterior disc this is back pain only, with a mid-disc it is back and leg pain, and with a lateral disc it is leg pain only. Acute disc prolapse is rarer in the cervical spine, but the classical picture is similar with radiation of pain to the arm rather than the leg.

Central disc prolapse is a rarer occurrence. Here the cord itself is pressed upon giving rise either to a paraplegia or a cauda equina lesion depending on the level—the cord finishes at L.1. It may also be the cause of narrowing of the spinal cord—spinal stenosis—which gives rise to symptoms called 'cord claudication'. One characteristic of this syndrome is the patient's ability to perform prolonged non-weight bearing exercise, such as cycling, while having restricted ability to perform weightbearing exercise, such as walking.

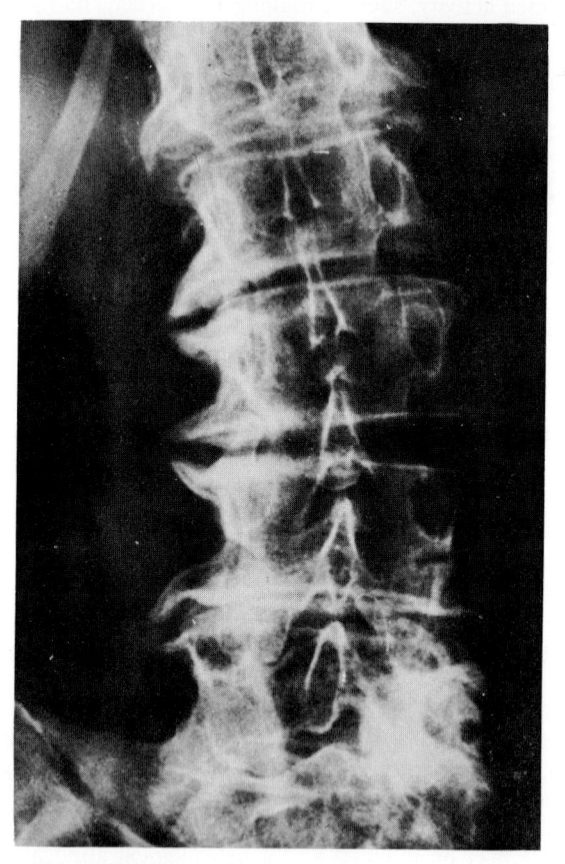

Fig. 7.6. Osteophytes from longstanding disc protrusion.

The majority of patients with spinal pain have less dramatic stories than those outlined above. Chronic dull pain in the low back is occasionally associated with radiation to the legs and buttocks but more frequently with pains up and down the length of the spine. These are not the product of nerve compression but of spasm in paraspinous muscles. The pain is frequently relieved by lying down, especially on a hard surface. Many patients relieve their discomfort by lying on the floor. Examination reveals alteration in the normal spinal curvature and diminished mobility which may be restricted to one or two directions of movement. Where lumbar articular derangement has occurred there may be a difference in side flexion on the side of the lesion. Unfortunately the physical signs elicited in lumbar spine disease often bear little relationship to the patient's symptoms.

Cervical spondylosis gives rise to similar symptoms, although pain radiating to the head, shoulders and arms is common even in the

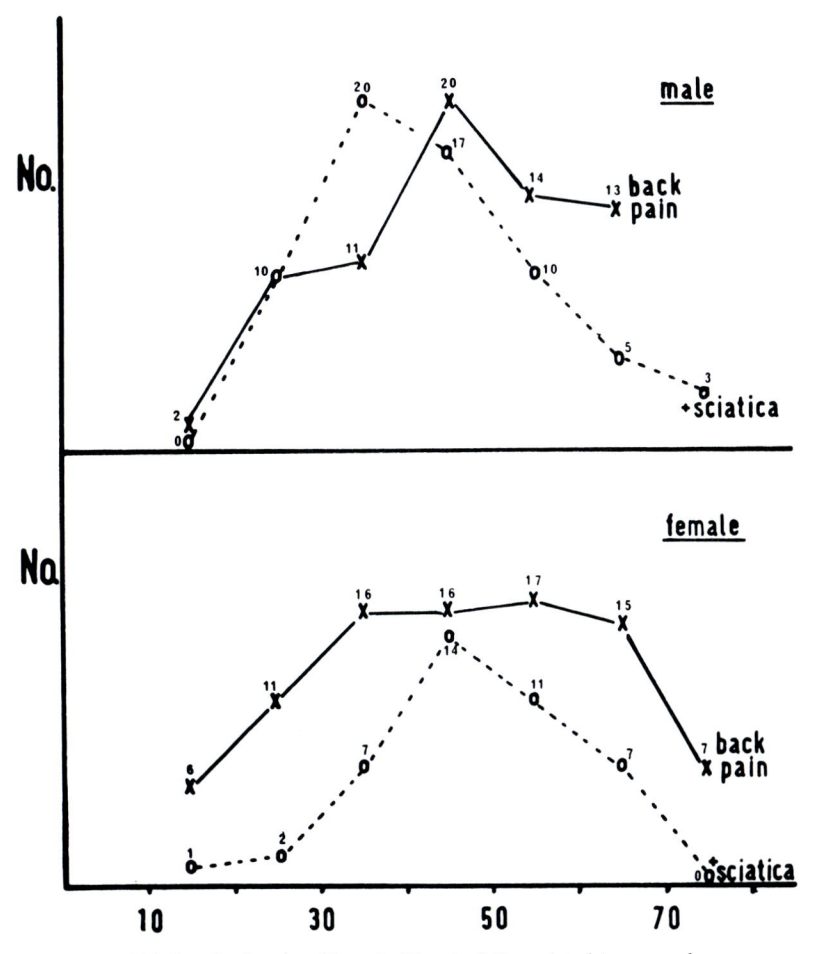

Fig. 7.7. Low back pain with and without sciatica related to age and sex.

absence of neurological signs. Movement is usually painful and night pain is a common feature. There may be a history of 'faints' on turning the head in one particular direction, due to osteophytes squeezing the vertebral arteries on their course to the brain. As in the lumbar spine the severity of the signs and symptoms may bear no relationship to each other.

Investigations

In general, investigations are unhelpful in degenerative spinal disease. There are no abnormal haematological or biochemical findings. Plain x-rays frequently show degenerative changes, but their position and extent does not bear a constant relationship to the patient's signs and symptoms. Exceptions to this are oblique views of the cervical spine, which may show osteophytes protruding into the intervertebral foramina from which the nerve roots emerge (Fig. 7.8), and oblique views

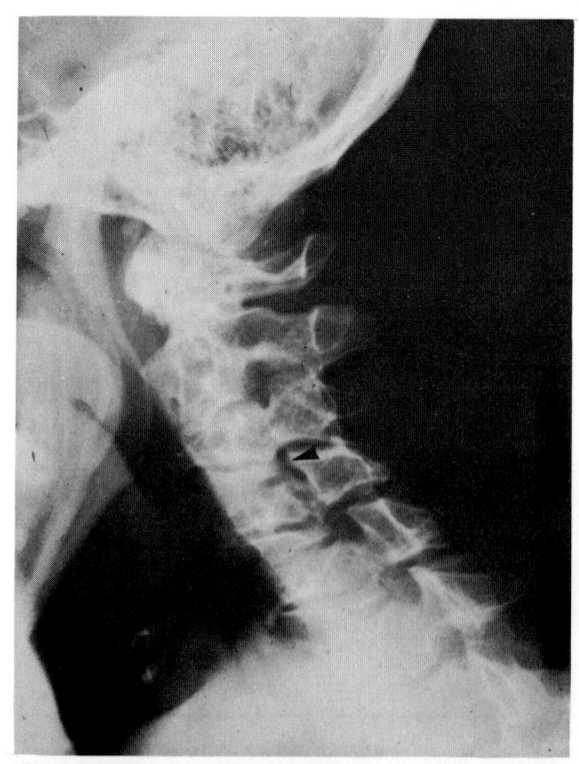

Fig. 7.8. Oblique x-ray of the cervical spine showing a narrowed foramen at the 3rd and 4th vertebrae.

of the lumbar spine which may show arthritis in the facet joints. These may also reveal defects in the vertebra which are associated with spondylolisthesis. Osteophytes may present a striking x-ray picture in the lumbar spine (Fig. 7.6).

In some patients the osteophytes may be very large and a condition of ankylosing hyperostosis occurs. In spondylolisthesis the defect in the vertebral arch allows a vertebra to slip forward on the one below due to lack of anchorage (Fig. 7.9). This may not be apparent on plain lateral

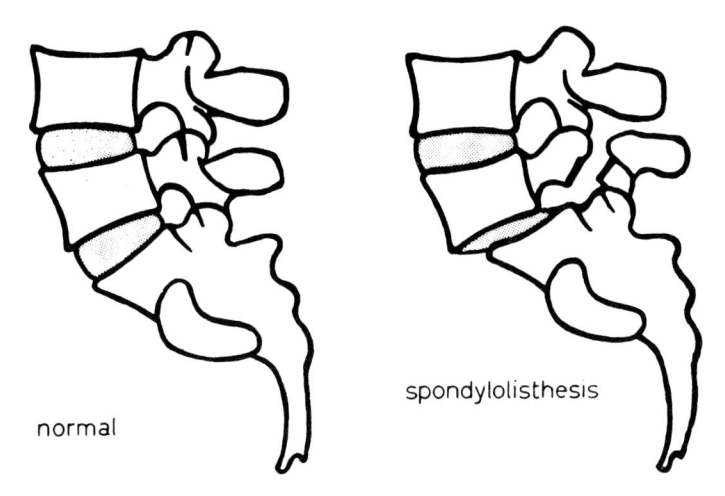

Fig. 7.9. Spondylolisthesis shown diagrammatically.

x-rays, but is sometimes detected by comparing the vertebral alignment on lying and standing films, where the forward slip may be detected.

Loss of calcium from the bone, osteoporosis, may be seen on plain x-rays. Measurement of the amount of calcium lost is not usually undertaken, but it must be remembered that about one third must be lost before osteoporosis can be detected on x-ray. Where osteoporosis is severe there may be collapse of the vertebrae, usually in the thoracic spine (Fig. 7.10). This may be an acute, dramatic event producing a sudden onset of pain in the thoracic spine with radiation in a girdle fashion around the body. More commonly it is found incidentally on the x-rays of the 'widow's hump' of elderly women or in patients on long-term steroid therapy.

Back symptoms appear to arise most commonly from the soft tissues of the spine—discs, ligaments and muscles. These are not seen on normal x-rays, but two techniques exist for investigating the discs. The most frequently performed is *myelography*. In this technique a lumbar puncture is performed, a few millilitres of spinal fluid removed, and a radio-opaque dye instilled instead. By tilting the patient the dye can be made to flow up and down the spinal canal. Protruding intervertebral discs can be seen as filling defects in the dye. This is a valuable pre-operative procedure as it allows the surgeon to plan which disc requires exposure at surgery. The second technique is *discography*,

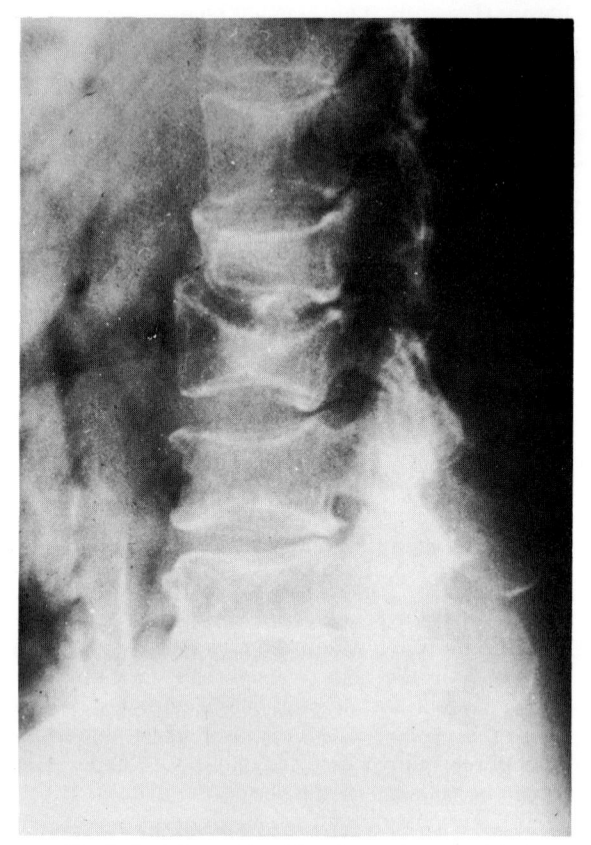

Fig. 7.10. Osteoporosis with collapse of vertebral body.

which is less widely used. A needle is inserted into the intervertebral disc and a small amount of radio-opaque dye injected. There are characteristic differences between the appearance of normal and abnormal discs, and the dye may outline a protrusion by flowing into it. The advantage of this procedure is that small protrusions are more easily seen. The main disadvantage is that every disc that is being investigated has to be punctured separately, as opposed to the single injection of myelography.

Treatment

Rest and traction

The cornerstone of treatment of acute disc prolapse is rest. The patient is initially rested in bed on a firm mattress or board. Analgesics and muscle relaxants, often with some sedation, are given to reduce the muscle spasm.

Where the symptoms are very acute, or there is no response to bed rest for a period of 10-14 days, the patient may be admitted to hospital for traction. Lumbar traction takes two forms. Pelvic traction is applied through a snugly fitting corset. This is attached by lateral tapes to a double pulley at the bed end. A single set of weights is used attached to both sides. Counterweight is applied by tipping the foot of the bed up and removing all the pillows. The advantage of this method is that it allows the patient's legs to be free, but it has the disadvantage of providing less strict immobilisation of the patient. The more widely used form of traction is skin traction. To apply this, the patient's legs are first shaved and Tincture Benzoin Co. is applied to the lateral and medial sides of the legs. One way stretch strapping with tapes stitched to the lower end is applied to each limb from the lateral malleolus on the lateral side to the greater trochanter and from the medial malleolus on the medial side to mid-thigh, the knee being kept straight. Three inch wide elastoplast is usually used, but narrower widths may suffice for a small or thin leg. While the plasters are being applied, small (approximately ¼ in.) nicks are cut with scissors in both upper and lower edges to ensure that the plaster is absolutely wrinkle free around the contours of the legs. With the more modern extension strapping lateral cuts are not required. The malleoli are then protected by sponge or orthopaedic felt and crepe bandages are applied from the malleoli upwards using 4 inch bandages to the knees and 6 inch bandages over the thighs. The tapes from each leg are passed through a spreader bar which is placed far enough below the foot to allow unimpeded plantar flexion to take place. The tapes are tied firmly at the far side of the spreader bar and traction cord is attached to the central hook of the spreader bar and passed over a pulley attached to the bottom end of the bed. An appropriate weight is then attached to each cord and the foot of the bed elevated. As with pelvic traction, the patient is nursed with no more than one pillow.

Patients must be warned to report symptoms arising from compression at the common peroneal nerve where it winds round the head of the fibula. The heels and Achilles tendon area are inspected regularly for pressure zones, and ankle mobility is maintained by frequent exercises. Calf muscle contractions must be undertaken to prevent deep venous thrombosis, and static quadriceps and hamstring muscle contractions minimise wasting. This form of traction provides better immobilisation at the expense of restriction of the legs, with the possibility of deep venous thrombosis, and some trauma to the patient when it is being removed.

Ventfoam traction is held to be kinder to the patient, but requires daily re-application in a similar fashion. The purpose of traction is not to pull the vertebrae apart, as this would require far more pull than that provided by the 10-24 lbs usually used. Traction provides good spinal rest and allows relaxation of the powerful paraspinous muscles and hence settling of the disc prolapse. In general, traction is applied until the patient has been asymptomatic for several days, and is then progressively withdrawn, the weights being taken off for a few hours more each day. Cervical traction is applied using a halter, the neck being supported in a neutral position and the head of the bed slightly elevated. Weights of 12-17 lbs are used. When traction fails to relieve the symptoms after three weeks, myelography is undertaken with a view to surgery being performed.

Physiotherapy

There are sharp differences of opinion regarding subsequent management. Different approaches include predominantly abdominal exercises, isometric back exercises or exercises including flexion or extension. Many patients are given a corset or plaster jacket for 3 to 6 months after coming off traction, the back muscles being re-educated at that time. Treatment of low back pain with various types of physiotherapy in one Scandinavian centre showed 85% improvement with traction, 60% with local heat and rest, and 45% with exercises. Cervical pain improved with exercises in 61%, with traction in 69% and with no treatment in 30%. The physician's assessment of improvement in this group was exercise 46%, traction 69% and no treatment 48%.

Treatment of the more chronic forms of backache is highly variable, the number of methods indicating the lack of efficacy of most of them. Most backache is self-limiting, and all claims of 'cures' must be examined with this in mind. Immobilisation is achieved by corsets or plaster jackets for the lumbar spine. A survey of over 3,000 patients in the USA showed the 51% preferred a corset, 34% a brace and 25% a cast. Collars of varying design have been used for the cervical spine. Plastazote is a particularly useful material for these. It is very

Degenerative Disease of the Spine

light—the weight of a cervical collar is that of an empty matchbox—and it can be made in the occupational therapy department. The material is mouldable at a hot, handleable temperature. Physiotherapy achieves muscle relaxation with radiant heat, short-wave diathermy or massage, coupled with intermittent traction applied mechanically to the back. In the neck manual or mechanical traction is used. Exercises may be given for the back and abdominal muscles. Mobilisation and manipulation may also be undertaken, but the most important part of the physiotherapist's treatment is advice on posture, lifting, working and sleeping positions (Figs. 7.11 & 7.12). The importance of this has

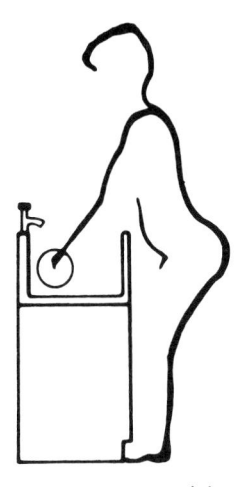

Fig. 7.11. Poor working posture: sink too low, no room for feet.

been demonstrated by direct pressure measurements taken in the L.3 disc while lifting, showing that the maximum pressure generated by lifting with the knees straight and the back bent is more than double that when the correct lifting posture—knees bent, back straight—is used. This is discussed in Chapter 15. The physiotherapist also demonstrates correct exercise for the spinal and abdominal muscles which can be carried out at home. Two useful books for patients are *You and Your Back* by David Delvin written for the Back Pain Association, and *Avoiding Back Trouble* by the Consumer's Association.

Drug therapy

Medical treatment includes the use of analgesics and muscle relaxants. Sleeping tablets are often needed and the combination of sedation and muscle relaxation makes diazepam 10 mg at night particularly valuable. Methocarbamol or baclofen may be taken during the day as they have no sedative effects. Extradural injection of corticosteroids may also be used either as an addition to traction, or to replace it, in acute disc prolapse. It is thought that some of the root symptoms are caused by inflammation around the nerve root rather than simple pressure of the

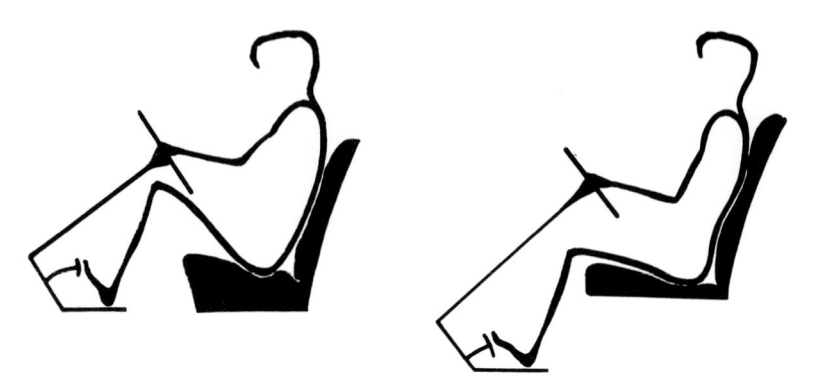

Fig. 7.12. Driving—bad and good postures. A) Poor seat for tall driver: no lumbar support, little leg room, seat too low. B) Relaxed driving position with good lumbar support and adequate seat height.

disc. Local corticosteroids may reduce this inflammation. The technique is similar to that of a lumbar puncture, although the sitting position, with the patient sitting on a chair with the legs straddling the seat and the face towards the chair back, is sometimes used. Using an aseptic technique a short-bevel needle is pressed forward until it is in the extradural space. If the dura is penetrated and CSF withdrawn the attempt must be abandoned. Methylprednisolone 80 mg is then injected, sometimes accompanied by 10 ml saline to aid distribution. Pain relief may be dramatic following this procedure. Where a single apophyseal joint appears to be the site of pain, intra-articular injection may be attempted using x-ray screening to follow the needle to the joint.

Where osteoporosis appears to be the cause of back pain, the logical treatment would be to replace the lost calcium. No method of doing this exists, but the use of calcium supplements, calcium and Vitamin D tablets, or calcium combined with anabolic steroids does provide symptomatic relief to some patients. Prevention of osteoporosis by hormone replacement therapy in menopausal women is becoming more widespread.

Surgery

This is indicated with lumbar disc protrusion if there is the sudden appearance or progression of neurological lesions. These may be muscle weakness or paralysis, or loss of sphincter control. Surgery may also be done if there is a failure to improve after 3 weeks rest in bed, or repeated attacks of pain after ambulation. In these circumstances excellent results are obtained in 38%, good in 41%, moderate in 18% and failure in 3%. It must be stressed, however, that surgery is not often needed. Of a group sufficiently severe to be admitted to hospital in Leeds, only 7% required surgery and half required bed rest only. On discharge, one quarter had no pain, 41% only mild pain and 57% no further time off work.

8
Non-articular Rheumatism

Trauma
Tenosynovitis
Dupuytren's Contracture
Bursitis
Epicondylitis
Carpal Tunnel Syndrome
Muscle Pain

Although the joints are the main organs affected by most rheumatic diseases, other structures of the body are also involved. Thus rheumatoid arthritis may involve other parts of the locomotor system, such as tendons and tendon sheaths, bones and muscles, as well as organs such as the heart, lungs and nerves. In some disorders, such as polymyositis, the main burden of the disease falls on a non-articular structure, the skeletal muscle in this example. Many patients, however, present to a rheumatological unit with musculo-skeletal symptoms which are not directly related to either 'joint' disease or the diffuse disorders of connective tissue. Many of these conditions are of uncertain cause and pathology. Lack of precise definition makes their study difficult. Most are selflimiting. Some of these conditions will be discussed in the section on painful feet (Chapter 13) e.g. plantar fasciitis, Achilles tendinitis and flat feet.

Trauma

A number of these disorders represent the effects of acute or chronic trauma. The sequence of events after a twisted ankle is familiar. Pain is rapidly followed by swelling, which may be severe, sometimes bruising and decreased function in the joint. In some patients, especially those in whom initial treatment was inadequate, the ankle may be 'weak' for the rest of their life. This 'weakness', usually reflected in a tendency to recurrent minor sprains as a result of trivial trauma, is not caused by ankle joint disease but by disruption of the peri-articular structures especially the ligaments. A similar sequence of events may occur in other parts of the body.

Tenosynovitis

Trauma may also predispose to inflammation in tendon sheaths and bursae. Tenosynovitis is an inflammation of tendon sheaths at any site in the body. It may occur as part of a generalised disease, such as rheumatoid arthritis, in some infective conditions (such as gonorrhoea and tuberculosis) or following repetitive trauma. Recently referred patients of our own with this condition have included a chicken catcher, a man who uses a compressed air gun and a keen badminton player. In each the extensor tendons of the wrist were painful on use and on forced extension. Redness and swelling of the tendon sheath occurs and rarely infection may supervene. In some cases movement of the tendon in the tendon sheath causes crepitus. De Quervain's tenosynovitis involves the extensor tendons of the thumb. Treatment is by avoiding the activity which caused the symptoms, rest (ideally in plaster of Paris) or local hydrocortisone injections. Occasionally surgery is required. 'Trigger finger' presents as an inability to extend the flexed finger without a sudden jerk (Fig. 8.1). It is due either to thickening of the flexor tendon sheaths or to a nodule in the tendon. The tendon and its sheath slip into the palm under the ligament across the metacarpal heads on flexing the finger. When the patient comes to straighten it however, the tight ligament prevents the tendon returning without a flick. The sudden extension gives rise to the name 'trigger finger'. The thickened sheath and tendon may be felt in the palm just proximal to the metacarpal head. Rheumatoid arthritis may cause this phenomenon, but it may also occur without a widespread arthritis. It is treated by local injection of corticosteroids. If injections on two or three occasions fail to relieve the condition, a small operation under local anaesthetic in which the ligament is divided cures it.

Dupuytren's Contracture

Thickening of the palmar fascia around the flexor tendons of the fingers produces flexion of the fingers. The condition was described by Baron Dupuytren, a French physician whom all living admired but few loved and no-one understood. The fascia binds down the skin in the palm, producing at first a small dimple. The little finger is usually the first to be pulled into flexion, followed by the ring finger and then the middle finger (Fig. 8.2). Under the microscope the tissue looks like a fibroma (a benign tumour), but it does not become malignant, nor does it have the general characteristics of a tumour. In some patients it is associated with alcoholism and/or cirrhosis of the liver. Dupuytren's first patient was a cooper, and Dupuytren attributed the condition to the pressure of the barrels he handled. It is now thought that the contents rather than the casks may have had more influence. Most patients have no obvious cause for the contracture. They tend to be in

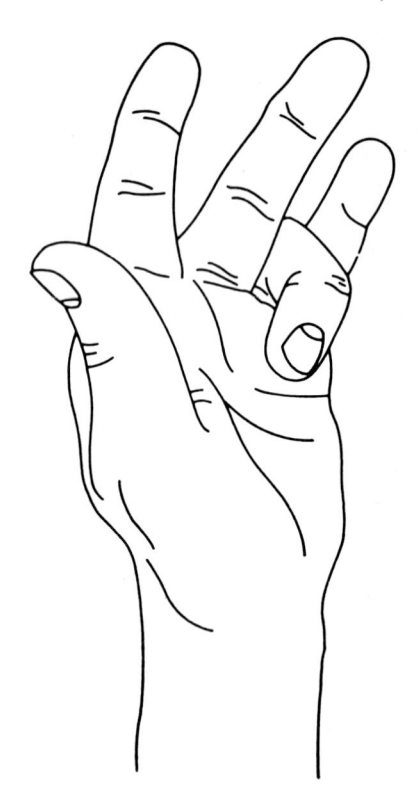

Fig. 8.1. Trigger finger.

the older age range (over 60 years), and the condition often runs in families. Many patients require no treatment for it. Others have the fascia removed by a plastic or an orthopaedic surgeon, but the operation is difficult. On rare occasions if the finger is bound tightly down and is troublesome either mechanically or because the patient cannot wash underneath it, the digit is amputated.

Bursitis

The pre-patellar bursa is inflamed in 'housemaid's knee'. 'Beat disease' in miners starts as a traumatic bursitis at the knees or elbows, although superadded infection or secondary osteoarthrosis may complicate the later stages. The use of knee and elbow pads by colliers has greatly reduced the incidence of this condition.

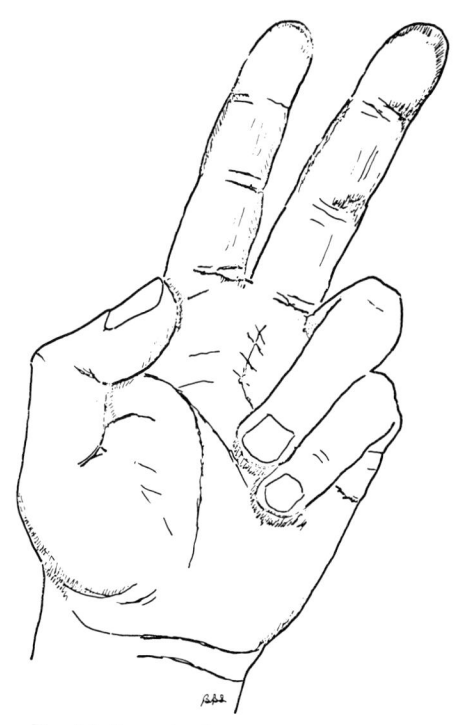

Fig. 8.2. Dupuytren's contracture.

Epicondylitis

'Tennis elbow', pain in the region of the lateral epicondyle of the elbow, is a common example of an overuse phenomenon. Although the exact pathology is unknown, a local inflammatory response probably follows tearing of some fibres in the common extensor origin. Corticosteroid injection is usually effective in relieving symptoms, though several injections may be needed. The condition occasionally becomes chronic. A similar syndrome at the medial epicondyle of the elbow is referred to as 'golfer's elbow'.

Carpal Tunnel Syndrome

The median nerve in the carpal tunnel may be compressed. This may occur as part of a generalised arthritis. 10% of patients with rheumatoid arthritis show the conditions. We have treated a number of patients whose first symptom of rheumatoid arthritis has been due to a carpal tunnel syndrome. Other patients have a disorder which produces thickening of surrounding tissue (such as myxoedema or acromegaly). Others have fluid retention (as in pregnancy) which compresses the nerve. The incidence in pregnant women is 7-18%, and it recovers after delivery. In many others, however, there is no known underlying cause. These are more often women, usually in their 40's or 50's.

The patient complains of pins and needles in the thumb, index, middle and half the ring fingers (i.e. the distribution of the median nerve). Symptoms are worst at night. They may waken the patient. Relief is gained by hanging the arm out of bed or shaking it. Pain and stiffness may also accompany the symptoms, and surprisingly the pain may radiate up the forearm. At a later stage the muscles of the ball of the thumb (thenar eminence) waste. The symptoms may be brought out by forcibly extending the wrist. These features are shown diagramatically in Fig. 8.3. Electrical tests of the nerve show that conduction of the nerve impulse is delayed. Both sides are involved in two-thirds of patients, with symptoms usually more marked on the right. The right side alone is affected in a quarter.

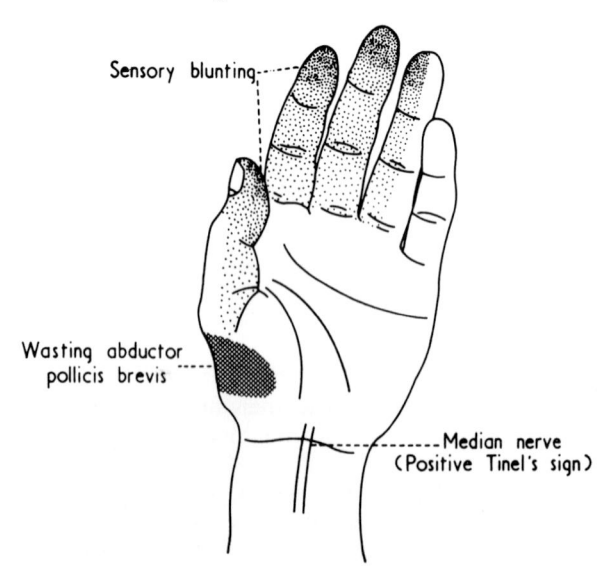

Fig. 8.3. Carpal tunnel syndrome.

Non-articular Rheumatism

Splintage of the wrist at night relieves symptoms. This may be a useful test where the diagnosis is in doubt. It is used in treatment during pregnancy, since the syndrome resolves after delivery. Diuretics have been given on the assumption that fluid retention is a factor in the condition, but they are not of proven use. Carpal tunnel decompression is the treatment of choice. It is a simple operation, usually done as a day case. If necessary it can be done under regional anaesthetic. Both carpal tunnels may be decompressed at the same operating session. This is not done if the patient lives alone, since both hands are bandaged for ten days.

Muscle Pain

Muscle pain may result from inflammation as part of a generalised disorder of connective tissue. Dermatomyositis is one example and will be discussed in Chapter 10. Weakness of the muscles may occur due to wasting (atrophy) from disuse of a joint. This may be caused by pain in the joint, or by limitation of movement from a bony or fibrous tissue block. Sometimes the muscle is affected by a disease without giving pain, e.g. myopathy in rheumatoid arthritis or from treatment with steroids.

In any pyrexial illness muscle aching may be prominent. Most of us are familiar with the generalised aching accompanying a viral infection. One particular virus (Coxsackie) may produce severe muscle pain. This is called epidemic myalgia or Bornholm disease. The pain may be around the chest and is often mistaken for pleurisy.

Pain related to muscles is a common feature of their use or overuse. Unusual exertion may cause severe stiffness and aching, but this decreases as use continues. Tears of muscle fibres are common athletic injuries and cause acute pain especially felt on movement. Rest allows healing, but some degree of support, for example an elastic calf support, may be needed during periods of exertion for months or years. Back pain following exertion is a universal phenomenon. Some patients complain of this because of an increasing expectation in some sections of the community that life should be painless and trouble-free from the cradle to the grave. Others use 'back pain' as a reason for not working. Many cases of acute and chronic back pain, however, arise from non-articular structures in the spine. Muscle spasm is often encountered and may be patchy, leading to the formation of 'fibrositis nodules'. On biopsy these small lumps in muscle simply consist of normal muscle fibres which were in spasm when felt.

The final group of patients with non-articular complaints does not have any obvious precipitating cause. These are the patients with 'muscular rheumatism', aches and pains felt mainly in muscles throughout the body, often worse in damp weather. Such pain may be the only symptom in thyroid deficiency. A small minority of these patients suffered from rheumatic fever in childhood, and such diffuse aching often becomes a chronic phenomenon in these patients. In many others no present or past cause can be found, and full physical, laboratory and x-ray examination reveals no causative abnormality. Some simply require reassurance that they have no crippling disease. Anxiety or tension contributes to the symptoms in many others. There is an unfortunate tendency for these patients to become chronic invalids partly because of their own anxiety and partly because of hesitation on the part of their doctors. They should be firmly told that they do not have arthritis and will not become cripples. They should be given only simple symptomatic treatment.

9

Shoulder Disorders

Anatomy
Rotator Cuff Disease
Subdeltoid Bursitis
Bicipital Tendinitis
Frozen Shoulder
Shoulder-hand Syndrome
Referred Pain

The joint between the humerus and the scapula, the gleno-humeral joint, may be involved as part of the generalised inflammatory diseases such as rheumatoid arthritis. Ankylosing spondylitis affects the shoulder in more than one-third of cases, though osteoarthrosis is uncommon in this non-weightbearing joint. The majority of shoulder disorders, however, are not due to specific arthritis in the gleno-humeral joint, but to less well defined conditions involving the whole shoulder girdle.

Anatomy

A knowledge of the anatomy of the shoulder region is essential if rheumatic disorders are to be understood (Figs. 9.1 & 9.2). There are three joints in the shoulder girdle, the gleno-humeral, acromio-clavicular and sterno-clavicular. In addition the gliding motion of the scapula across the back of the rib cage makes it the functional equivalent of a joint. Although each of these has isolated functions, normal shoulder movements involve them all.

The gleno-humeral joint is a very shallow ball-and-socket type. Stability of the joint has been sacrificed in order to give a wide range of movement. The stability of the joint is maintained by the surrounding muscles and tendons. The insertions of the supraspinatus, infraspinatus, teres minor and subscapularis are collectively called the rotator cuff. Between the insertion of the cuff and the deltoid lies the subdeltoid bursa. The other significant structure is the long head of

90 Rheumatism for Nurses & Remedial Therapists

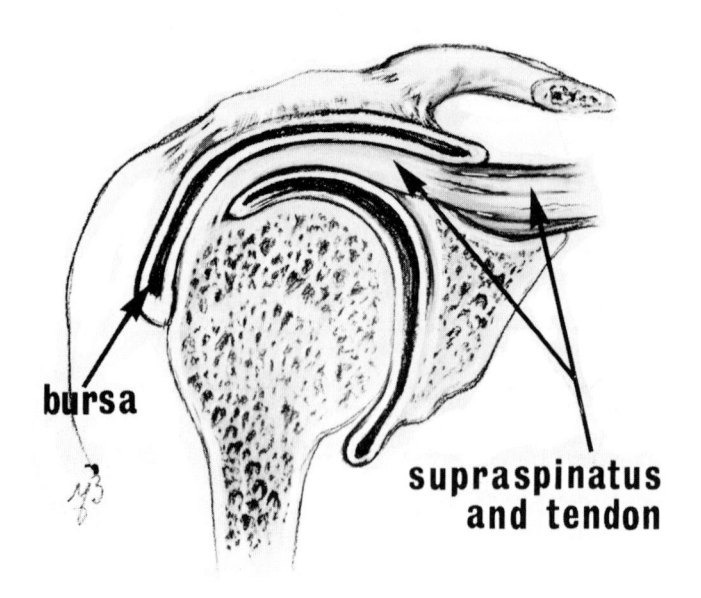

Fig. 9.1. Anatomy of shoulder joint, showing supraspinatus tendon and subacromial bursa.

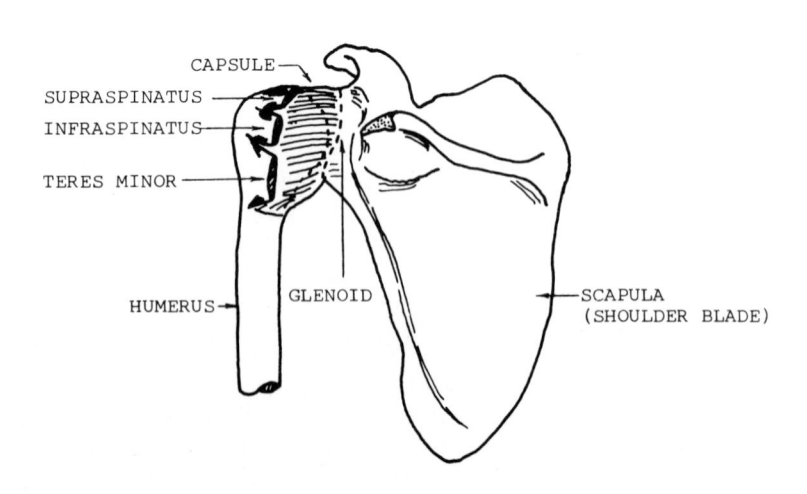

Fig. 9.2. Shoulder joint from behind.

biceps which travels up the bicipital groove in the humerus to be inserted into the scapula above the glenoid margin.

Rotator Cuff Disease

The tendons forming the rotator cuff are particularly liable to degeneration. This may lead to calcification in the supraspinatus tendon or rupture of one or more of the tendons forming the cuff. The subdeltoid bursa is often secondarily inflamed. Occasionally a calcific lesion bursts and extrudes material into the bursa (Fig. 9.3). This

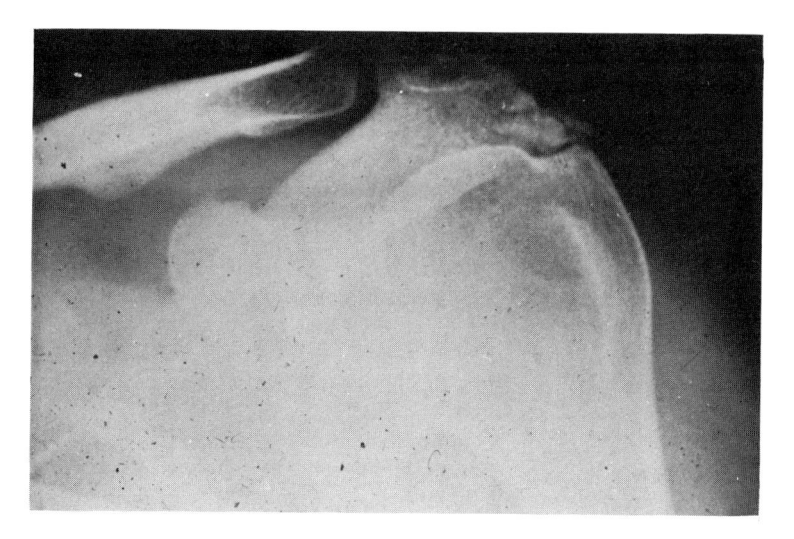

Fig. 9.3. Calcification in a subacromial bursa.

causes a severe reactive bursitis. Lesions of the cuff cause pain and restriction in movement of the shoulder which may take the form of a 'painful arc'. This is typically associated with calcific tendinitis, and comprises an initial pain-free range of abduction, a painful middle third of that movement followed by a painless completion of it.

Treatment is by rest during the acute phase, local infiltration of hydrocortisone into the affected area and appropriate exercises, physiotherapy being the more important measure. Repair of ruptured tendons is usually impractical due to the degenerative nature of the condition.

Subdeltoid Bursitis

This may occur as an isolated incident but is usually the result of cuff lesions which should be treated in parallel with it.

Bicipital Tendinitis

This is less common. Inflammation occurs in the isolated synovial sheath which surrounds the tendon in the bicipital groove. Fortunately the condition is usually self-limiting as treatment with local corticosteroids, rest or exercises gives unpredictable results.

Frozen Shoulder

This is a blanket term applied to painful, stiff shoulders. It is sometimes termed 'periarthritis of the shoulder'. Attempts have been made to separate different groups of patients, but the result appears to be the same whether degenerative, inflammatory or traumatic lesions are the precipitating cause. It usually begins between the ages of 40 and 60 years. Women are somewhat more often affected than men—in a study of 186 patients we did, the sex ratio was female:male 3:2. The pain was usually gradual in onset and of moderate severity. Sometimes, however, it would keep the patient awake at night, especially in the early stages. It often radiated down the outer aspect of the arm to the elbow and occasionally to the hands and fingers. Pain from the gleno-humeral joint tends to be felt over the deltoid region, that from other structures over the tip of the shoulder (Fig. 9.4).

In our series most of the men were manual workers. The disease occurred more commonly between the months of October to April than between the months of May to September. The majority of patients had unilateral involvement (70%). A history of trauma precipitating the condition was given in 2.8% of the men and 3.6% of the women. Psychological assessment showed that the periarthritic patients tended to worry more than a control group—this was particularly true amongst the women, and they suffered from insomnia more frequently than the control group before the periarthritis began. These differences were not statistically significant. Using sophisticated ways of measuring neuroticism and extroversion we could find no difference between the patients with periarthritis of the shoulder and other people. There was frequently a previous history of 'rheumatism' prior to the episode of periarthritis. In a third of the women 'non-specific rheumatism' had occurred. Cervico-brachial pain and a previous episode of shoulder pain had occurred more often in the women.

On clinical examination it was common to find tenderness over the bicipital groove, over the subacromial region and in the surrounding muscles. There was no significant anaemia. A mildly raised sedimentation rate was found in 14%. A mild leucocytosis was found in 14% of the men and none of the women.

Degenerative changes were found at the gleno-humeral joint in 6 to 9%, and at the acromio-clavicular joint in 31% of the men and 44% of

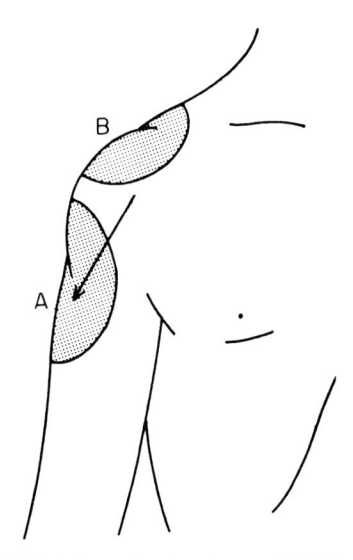

Fig. 9.4. Pain from the gleno-humeral joint is felt in the region of the deltoid insertion (A). Pain from other structures of the shoulder-girdle is generally referred to the point of the shoulder (B).

the women. Calcification was found around 11 of the shoulder joints.

In general this condition lasts for no longer than two years. As with all self-limiting conditions, extravagant claims are made for pet forms of treatment, all of which are successful as the disease will eventually improve spontaneously. Symptomatic relief with analgesics, an appropriate hypnotic if sleep is disturbed and judicious exercise make the waiting time for natural recovery more tolerable and may hasten it.

Controlled trials of treatments comprising hydrocortisone to the joint and exercises, hydrocortisone to the bicipital tendon and exercises, heat and exercises, were compared with analgesics alone. The treatment groups did better than the group who received only analgesics, but no one treatment was better than the other. The maximum effect was gained within three weeks.

Shoulder-hand Syndrome

The combination of a painful stiff shoulder with changes in the hand is known as the shoulder-hand syndrome. The hand becomes swollen with tight-looking, shiny skin. Hair may be lost from the hand, which loses the ability to sweat. The thickened fingers fail to function and become stiff and painful. Palmar thickening similar to Dupuytren's contractures may occur. X-rays show spotty osteoporosis in the bones. The time-course of the disease is shown in Fig. 9.5.

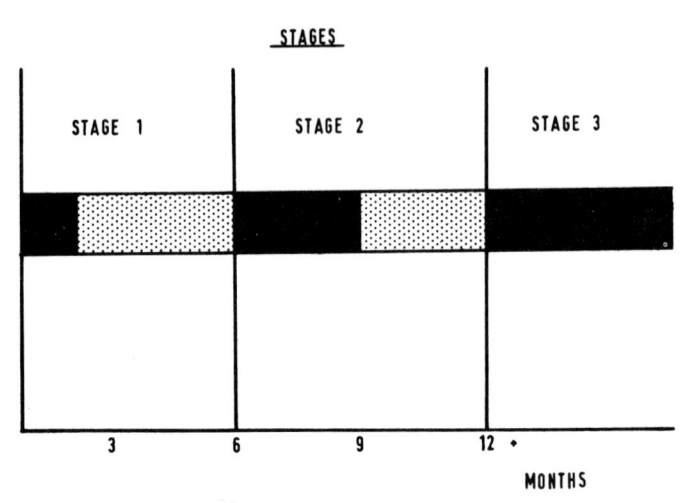

Fig. 9.5. The time-course of the shoulder-hand syndrome. The shaded areas represent the patients who do not progress to the next stage.

Shoulder-hand syndrome follows a variety of disorders of the limb including hemiplegia, acute inflammatory lesions of the hand or shoulder, myocardial infarction or trauma. The associated conditions in 220 patients are shown in Fig. 9.6. Treatment should be vigorous or severe handicap may result. Physical therapy should concentrate on maintaining both shoulder and hand function independently. Oral prednisolone appears to improve the recovery.

Referred Pain

As well as disease in the shoulder girdle, shoulder pain may be produced by reference from distant structures. Pain in the neck is often associated with shoulder or arm pain either from pressure on the nerve roots or from spasm in the neck muscles. Both shoulder and neck pain

Shoulder Disorders

are often associated with psychological features such as anxiety, insomnia and depression. The term 'periarthritic personality' is sometimes applied to those patients with cervico-brachial pain. This is sometimes less kindly expressed as 'people with pain in the neck are pains in the neck'.

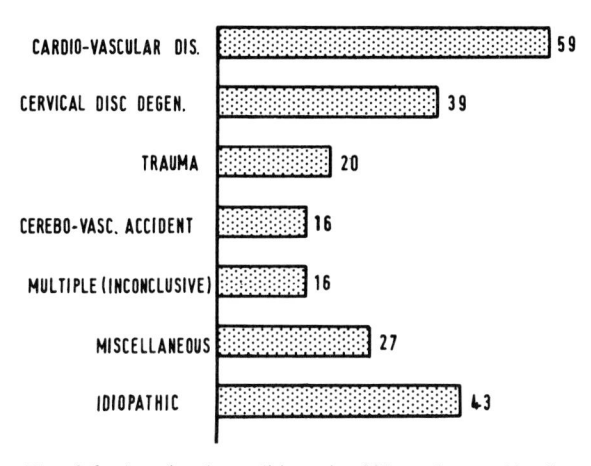

CARDIO-VASCULAR DIS.	59
CERVICAL DISC DEGEN.	39
TRAUMA	20
CEREBO-VASC. ACCIDENT	16
MULTIPLE (INCONCLUSIVE)	16
MISCELLANEOUS	27
IDIOPATHIC	43

Fig. 9.6. Associated conditions in 220 patients with the shoulder-hand syndrome.

More distant reference may be from structures in the chest, such as the typical radiation of pain from angina or myocardial infarction. Apical carcinoma of the lung, the Pancoast tumour, may present with shoulder pain. Reference may also be from disease adjacent to the diaphragm, such as subphrenic abscess, as the phrenic nerve is derived from cervical 4 and 5 segments of the spinal cord and has an area of skin reference over the shoulder. The shoulder pain caused by these conditions is only relieved when the underlying disease is controlled.

10

The Diffuse Connective Tissue Diseases

Systemic Lupus Erythematosus
  Aetiology
  Clinical features
  Laboratory tests
  Treatment
  Drug induced SLE
  Prognosis
Systemic Sclerosis
  Aetiology
  Clinical features
  Laboratory tests
  Treatment
  Prognosis
Polymyositis and Dermatomyositis
  Clinical features
  Laboratory tests
  Treatment
Polyarteritis Nodosa
  Clinical features
  Laboratory tests
  Treatment

This group of diseases, formerly called the 'Collagen Diseases', gain their name from the fact that connective tissue throughout the body may be affected by them. Their effects are widespread, and the involvement of many organ systems means that they are encountered in many medical and surgical specialties. They are also of great interest to laboratory workers, especially immunologists, because of the wide variety of alterations in laboratory tests which they cause.

Although the diseases will be discussed separately, it must be remembered that each of these conditions shows considerable overlap

The Diffuse Connective Tissue Diseases

with other members of the group, i.e. some features thought to be characteristic of one disease may be found in patients suffering from another.

Systemic Lupus Erythematosus (SLE)

This disease occurs mainly in women, and usually starts during childbearing years (Fig. 10.1). It is characterised by involvement of many organ systems throughout the body, but not all the manifestations occur in any one patient.

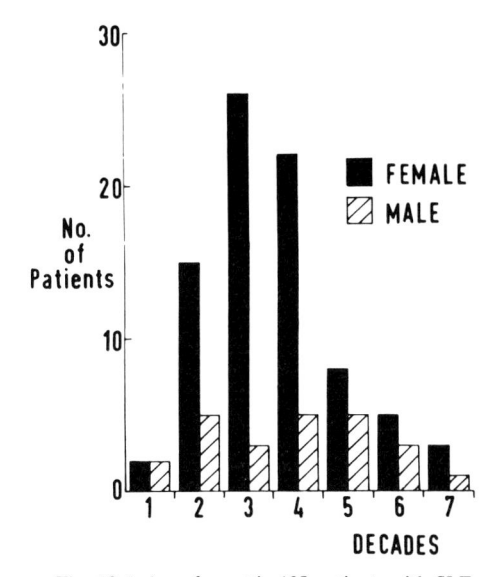

Fig. 10.1. Age of onset in 105 patients with SLE.

Aetiology

The cause of SLE is unknown. Recent research has suggested that viruses may be involved in some way in causing the disease, but this is not certain. Many abnormalities of the immune system in the body occur during the course of the disease. It has, therefore, been suggested that this is an 'auto-immune' disease, that is one in which normal immunological defence mechanisms turn on the patient's own body and react to it as if it were a foreign invader. Some drugs may cause a lupus-like disease (see below). The incidence of SLE seems to be increasing, especially in the USA where there is a relatively high incidence in the negro population.

Clinical features

The most common presentation of the disease is with arthralgia (pain in the joints) which may be accompanied by fever. The joints may be warm and red, but the symptoms suffered by the patient often seem excessive in comparison to the physical signs found in the joints. The pattern of joint involvement is similar to that seen in rheumatoid arthritis, and morning stiffness is a prominent feature. In contrast to rheumatoid arthritis, the joints of patients with SLE do not develop destructive changes or severe deformity despite years of joint symptoms.

Fever is a common feature of SLE both at presentation and during exacerbation of the disease. One of the most characteristic features of the disease is the rash which occurs in almost all patients at some stage. The classical rash is in a 'butterfly' distribution over the face, the 'wings' spreading over the upper part of the cheeks. This occurs in about half the patients, the rest showing variable types of rash usually involving exposed areas of the body and often precipitated by sunlight (solar dermatitis). The form of these lesions is very variable, from erythematous lesions to urticaria. Erythematous lesions at the finger tips and around the nail base are often seen, especially in acute cases and similar lesions may appear on the palms. Raynaud's phenomenon is a common finding, in which the fingers go cold, dead and white in the cold. The scalp is affected and either patchy alopecia (baldness) or a characteristic bunch of broken hairs over the forehead may appear. The skin lesions vary in duration from transient rashes, often following exposure to sunlight, to chronic eruptions.

Patients with SLE are often generally ill with malaise, anaemia, weight loss and a tendency to fatigue. Muscle wasting may occur, especially round joints.

Involvement of the kidneys occurs in about one-third of patients with SLE. The patient's prognosis is closely linked with the presence of renal disease and the histological type of the involvement. The first evidence of renal involvement may be proteinuria or haematuria. Careful urine testing is important in the management of patients with SLE as the treatment depends on early identification of the type of renal damage. This differentiation is made by needle biopsy of the kidney, a procedure which may be required on several occasions to assess the progress of the renal disease.

Inflammation of serous membranes occurs throughout the body giving rise to pericarditis or pleurisy with or without effusion. Inflammation of the peritoneum is one of the 'medical' causes of the acute abdomen, and great care must be taken not to allow lupus patients presenting with abdominal pain to become dehydrated, as this may increase their renal damage.

The Diffuse Connective Tissue Diseases

Not only the pericardium but the other layers of the heart may be involved in SLE. Myocarditis and endocarditis are rarely the cause of severe disability, although the characteristic Libman-Sacks vegetations may be found on the heart valves at post-mortem examination (these are small, compact, pale, adherent, irregular outgrowths). More serious involvement of the cardiovascular system takes the form of vasculitis. Inflammation usually involves the walls of small arteries, although larger arteries are occasionally involved. Vasculitis may lead to gangrene of the finger tips. Arteritis in the gut may cause functional disturbance or even gangrene of the bowel. Punched out ulcers in the legs may also be a manifestation of vasculitis.

Enlargement of lymph nodes occurs in about half the patients with SLE and may be sufficiently severe to arouse the clinical suspicion of a lymphoma. The liver is enlarged in about one third of patients, though this is rarely of clinical importance. Splenomegaly, which in the past was thought to be of considerable diagnostic importance, is in fact found in less than one quarter of patients.

The impact of SLE on the nervous system is being increasingly recognised. Peripheral neuropathy is fairly rare, but central involvement including fits may be seen. Psychiatric disturbance occurs frequently, varying from irritability to paranoia. These disturbances usually accompany a generalised exacerbation of the disease, but new more sensitive diagnostic tests for SLE have shown that some patients have a psychiatric disturbance as the only clinical sign of the disease.

Laboratory tests

The clinical diagnosis of SLE may be difficult, as the disease may present clinically with any or all of the above symptoms and signs. In these circumstances blood tests may be of great value. These are listed:
 ESR high (often more than 100 mm 1st hour)
 Gamma globulin high
 Immunoglobulins altered
 LE cells
 Anti-nuclear antibodies
 DNA antibodies (may help early detection of exacerbations).
These are further discussed in Chapter 19.

Treatment

The skin disease may be helped by avoiding exposure to sunlight or by the use of corticosteroid creams. Antimalarial drugs, such as chloroquine, are also used. Symptoms from the joints may be controlled by analgesic/anti-inflammatory medication of the aspirin type. The systemic part of the disease is usually controlled by corticosteroids which may need to be given in very high doses during acute exacerbations of the disease. Renal disease may require the use of cytotoxic agents such as cyclophosphamide or azathioprine for its control.

Drug induced SLE

Some drugs are known to precipitate an illness very similar to SLE. The joint disease is very similar, but the systemic part of the disease is usually less severe, and renal and central nervous system involvement are never prominent. LE cells and anti-nuclear factor are found in the blood, and the ESR is raised.

Drugs producing this include procainamide, hydrallazine, phenytoin, oral contraceptives and anti-bacterial agents such as sulphonamides, penicillins, streptomycin and tetracycline. Many other drugs have caused this condition on rare occasions.

Treatment is by withdrawing the drug, which is always followed by rapid resolution of the disease.

Prognosis

The outlook for this disease was at one time thought to be generally serious. This is well shown in Fig. 10.2, where over a period of nearly 25 years the mortality of SLE in the literature has fallen from 100% to 26%. This is due in small measure to more effective treatment, for instance with steroids, but is largely due to the recognition of milder forms of the disease. If the kidney is involved, this is a serious sign.

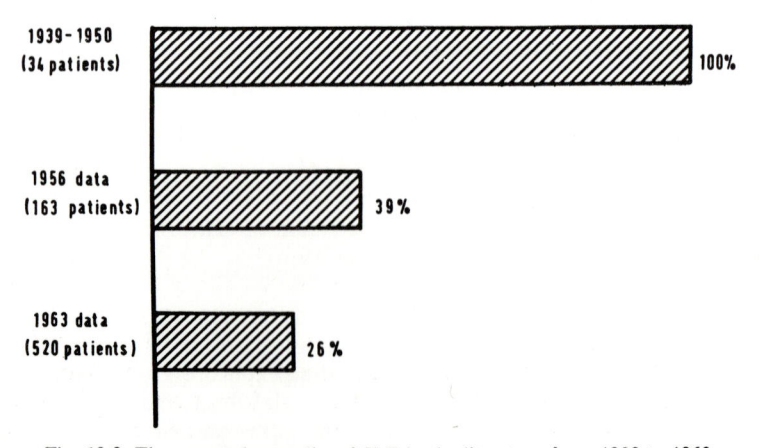

Fig. 10.2. The reported mortality of SLE in the literature from 1939 to 1963.

When the disease is induced by drugs, withdrawal of the offending agent produces recovery in the patient. Intercurrent infection should be treated quickly and vigorously, as this may kill the patient.

Systemic Sclerosis

This name is now preferred to scleroderma as it highlights the generalised nature of the disease. As the name implies, in this disease there is thickening of connective tissue throughout the body.

Aetiology

The cause of systemic sclerosis is unknown. It is twice as common in women as men and, like SLE, appears to be more common in American negroes.

Clinical features

These may vary from localised areas of sclerosis in the skin to a progressive disorder with widespread effects leading to death.

The skin lesions start with oedema which progresses to a characteristic thickening and tightening of the skin. In patients in whom the disease appears to be confined to the skin small areas of thickened skin called linear morphoea may be the only visible evidence of disease. When the generalised disease occurs, however, the fingers are most commonly involved, becoming tight, hard and shiny. Involvement of the face gives rise to a characteristic 'presbyterian' expression, with a tight, puckered, disapproving mouth which cannot be opened fully. Telangiectasia, the appearance of tiny red lines caused by dilated capillaries and minute arterioles, and alterations in pigmentation, both local depigmentation and more generalised hyperpigmentation, may occur.

Raynaud's phenomenon is common early in the course of the disease, but more serious evidence of decreased blood supply becomes apparent as the disease progresses. These include ulceration and gangrene of the fingers and 'whittling down' of the terminal phalanges. Occasionally auto-amputation of digits occurs.

Soft tissue calcification occurs in about 10% of patients (Fig. 10.3). Calcific deposits under the skin may cause overlying ulceration, with extrusion of the calcific material. The synovium of joints may be calcified, but joint involvement is more usually felt as pain and stiffness in the affected joints, usually the small joints of the hands. A destructive arthritis does not occur. Although joint swelling may occur, this is often made to appear worse by the tightness of the surrounding skin.

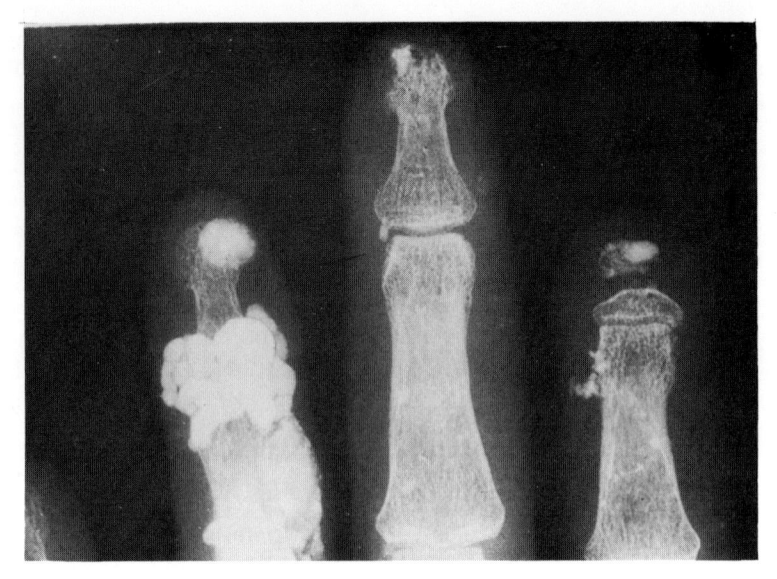

Fig. 10.3. Calcinosis around a digit in scleroderma.

Involvement of tendon sheaths by the thickening process occurs quite commonly. Involved tendons may be creaky and painful. Myopathy may occur, involved muscles showing tenderness and wasting.

The gut is extensively involved in systemic sclerosis. The best recognised defect is in the oesophagus, which loses its normal motility and becomes a wide immobile tube. This gives rise to difficulty in swallowing, and sometimes to 'overspill pneumonitis' in which the stagnant contents of the dilated oesophagus spill over into the lungs causing inflammation. Similar abnormalities are now recognised in the small intestine, where loss of normal peristalsis may lead to stagnation. This is often accompanied by abdominal distension. In the bowel, wide mouthed diverticulae or outpouchings are produced.

As well as being involved by overspill pneumonitis, the lungs may also be the site of inflammatory changes and thickening of the alveolar walls leading to pulmonary fibrosis.

Laboratory tests

There is no diagnostic test for systemic sclerosis, but abnormalities found include a moderately raised ESR and the presence of rheumatoid factor and antinuclear factor in the blood.

X-rays may show calcification in the hand and whittling away of the tips of the terminal phalanges, the 'peg top' appearance.

The Diffuse Connective Tissue Diseases

Treatment

In general the treatment of systemic sclerosis is very unsatisfactory. Many therapies have been suggested which either affect inflammation or alter the metabolism of collagen. None has been shown to alter the prognosis in this disease, although the natural variations which occur in the severity of the disease often leads to extravagant claims of 'cures'. No cure exists. Some improvement in the stiffness of hands may occur as a result of exercise in oil baths. Deep connective massage has also been advocated.

Prognosis

Scleroderma confined to the skin carries no threat to life, but with more widespread involvement the condition may be fatal (Fig. 10.4). The

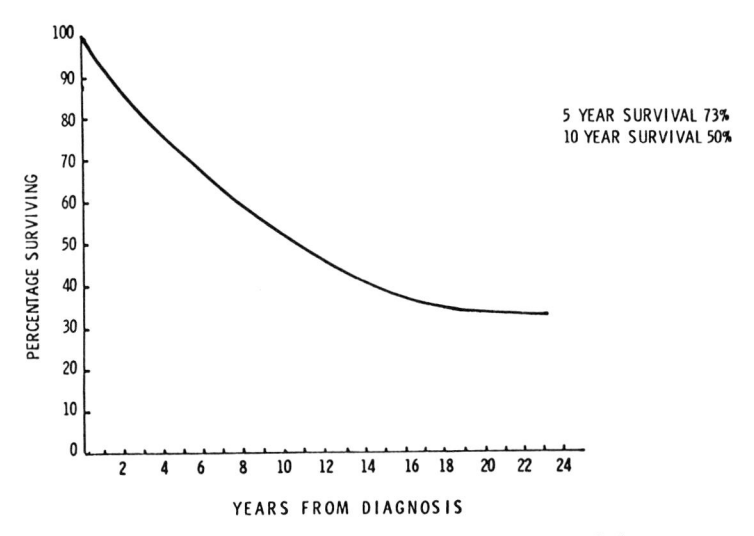

Fig. 10.4. Survival in scleroderma over a 23-year period.

five-year survival is 73.8%; the ten-year survival is 50%. The outlook is poorer, when lung changes occur, when the kidney is affected giving a raised blood urea, when there are abnormalities of the electrocardiograph and when the trunk is involved.

Polymyositis and Dermatomyositis

These are conditions in which widespread inflammatory changes occur in skeletal muscle. Where the disease is restricted to muscle the term polymyositis is used. Where skin changes also occur the disease is called dermatomyositis. The disease is rare. It can occur at any age from childhood to senescence, but is most common in the 30 to 60 age group. Women are affected about twice as often as men. A classification of polymyositis, devised by Professor Walton of Newcastle, is shown in Table 10.1.

1.	Pure polymyositis
2.	Polymyositis with minor features of other connective tissue disorders or a slight rash
3.	Other connective tissue disorders with incidental polymyositis

4.	Dermatomyositis
	    A. Adult — with malignancy
	              — without malignancy
	    B. Childhood

Table 10.1 Classification of Polymyositis.

Clinical features

The disease usually presents as a slow onset of muscular weakness and wasting. This is often symmetrical and tends to affect proximal muscle groups first. The involved muscles may be tender and there is sometimes brawny oedema over them. Muscle biopsies show extensive inflammatory change with destruction of muscle fibres.

The rash of dermatomyositis is usually described as a heliotrope discolouration, that is it is erythematous with pale purple overtones. This often occurs around the eyes and is associated with oedema, but may spread over the whole face. Erythematous lesions also occur over the 'shawl area' of the shoulders, and on the fingers, where they may form linear streaks.

Arthritis occurs in more than a third of patients, and is similar to the symmetrical, non-destructive joint involvement found in other connective tissue diseases.

About half the patients with dermatomyositis presenting over the age of 55 have an underlying cancer. The most common sites are the ovary, lung, breast and stomach. Most patients in this age group will, therefore, need to be investigated thoroughly to exclude these cancers, though in younger patients such investigations are usually restricted to those who fail to respond to treatment.

Laboratory tests

Apart from tests done during the search for an underlying cancer, a rise may occur in the ESR and rheumatoid factor or antinuclear factor may appear in the blood. Muscle destruction is accompanied by the release of muscle enzymes, such as creatine phosphokinase, which may be present in abnormal amounts. Electromyography shows the presence of muscle damage, though the changes are not diagnostic, and muscle biopsy may be undertaken.

Treatment

Corticosteroids often control the inflammation, but need to be given in high doses starting at 60 mg prednisolone daily in acute cases. Maintenance doses are usually in the range 10-15 mg prednisolone daily. Where no response occurs a search for an underlying cancer is undertaken, as removal usually produces improvement in the muscle and skin diseases. Cytotoxic agents have been used in patients who have failed to respond to corticosteroids.

Polyarteritis Nodosa

In this rare disease the inflammation affects the walls of arteries, mainly those of medium size, but spreads to involve small and, occasionally, large vessels. The inflammation often leads to thrombosis occurring in the artery and the symptoms and signs produced are, therefore, those of loss of blood supply to the affected part.

Clinical features

Although the clinical features may be very widespread, the typical onset is with a vague generalised illness with malaise, pyrexia, weakness and weight loss. The kidneys are usually involved and urine testing shows haematuria or proteinuria. Involvement of renal vessels may lead either to renal failure or to the development of hypertension.
    Peripheral neuropathy occurs because the vessels in the nerve sheath, the vasi nervori, may be involved leading to death of nerve fibres. Heart failure may follow the development of hypertension or myocardial infarction produced by arteritis rather than the usual coronary atheroma. Many patients have alterations in gastro-intestinal function because of the poor blood supply to the gut. There may be abdominal pain and distension, malabsorption or ulceration of the gut. Gangrene may occur. Joint pains and swelling are quite common and other organ systems are involved more rarely.
    In general the prognosis is poor, most patients dying from kidney or heart involvement.

Laboratory tests

There are no diagnostic tests, but anaemia, a high ESR and biochemical changes due to renal failure may be seen. Some patients show high levels of eosinophils in their blood. Rheumatoid factor is present in some patients. The diagnosis is usually established by biopsy of an affected part, kidney or muscle biopsies being the most usual.

Treatment

High doses of corticosteroids are used, usually starting with 60 mg prednisolone daily and reducing to a maintenance dose of 10-20 mg daily.

11

Rheumatic Fever

Aetiology
Pathology
Clinical Features
Investigations
Differential Diagnosis
Treatment
Sequelae

Rheumatic fever, called 'acute rheumatism', is a group of clinical conditions caused by β haemolytic streptococcus infection. The term 'group of clinical conditions' is used because this disease may manifest itself in many ways. The diagnostic criteria proposed by the American Heart Association are shown in Table 11.1—at least one major and two minor criteria are required to make a diagnosis. Its importance lies not only in the recognition and treatment of the acute disease but also in its long term effects which are frequently of more importance.

Aetiology

Many studies have shown that infection with β haemolytic streptococci is the essential starting point of rheumatic fever. It is equally clear that the various manifestations of the disease are not caused by direct infection by these organisms. As the disease only follows a small minority of streptococcal infections, estimated as less than 3% of cases of untreated streptococcal pharyngitis, it seems likely that the production of the disease is caused by an abnormality in the body's response to the invading streptococci. The nature of this abnormal reaction is, at present, unknown. The sequence of events is shown diagrammatically in Fig. 11.1. The incidence of rheumatic fever has fallen markedly this century. The reasons for this are not completely understood. The widespread use of penicillin, to which the streptococcus has never acquired resistance, in treating sore throats has been a contributing factor.

Major	Minor

Carditis
Polyarthritis
Chorea
Nodules
Erythema
   marginatum
	ESR raised
	PR interval increased on ECG
	Recent streptococcal infection
	Reliable history of rheumatic fever or evidence
	   of pre-existing rheumatic heart disease

Table 11.1 Diagnostic criteria of rheumatic fever proposed by the American Heart Association. One major and two minor criteria are required for the diagnosis.

Rheumatic fever has always been most widespread in poor social conditions, especially crowded houses, and social improvements have also played a part. It also seems likely that some change has taken place in the streptococcus which has made it less likely to initiate rheumatic fever. In considering past information regarding rheumatic fever it must be remembered that the definition of what constitutes the disease varies from author to author, so that direct comparisons of different studies cannot be made in may cases. In particular when acute rheumatism was more widespread and more feared, any acute arthritis in childhood, and even 'growing pains', were likely to be considered as rheumatic fever and the child treated accordingly. It is probable that many children who have never suffered from this disease have had their lives unnecessarily restricted in the past.

Pathology

Studies of the pathology of rheumatic fever are biased in two ways. Firstly, the patients dying during the course of the acute disease

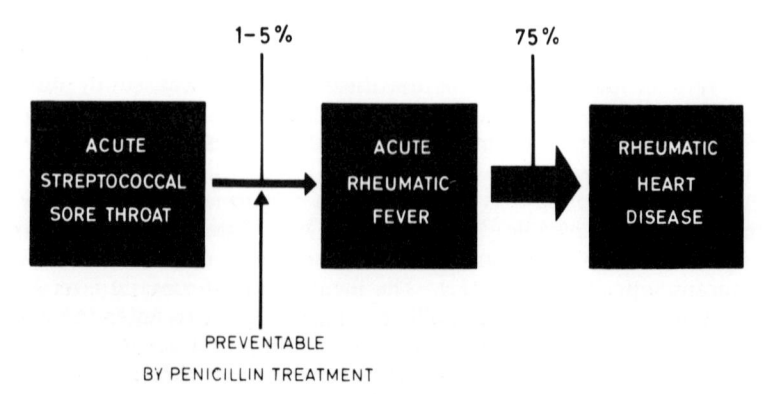

Fig. 11.1. Aetiology of rheumatic heart disease.

represent a small minority of the total number of cases seen. By definition this minority is drawn from the most severe part of the disease spectrum. Secondly the patients dying in the acute phase almost always do so because of heart disease. This means that post mortem series exaggerate the importance of cardiac damage in the general population of patients with the disease.

The pathological changes seen in the heart vary according to the duration of the disease. Death during the acute phase is caused by myocarditis. The heart muscle appears soft and flabby, and histology shows an inflammatory infiltration of the myocardium with destruction of the muscle cells. Characteristic lesions called Aschoff's nodes (or Aschoff's bodies) may be seen in the myocardium. These consist of an accumulation of inflammatory cells in a loose cluster around a centre of degenerating muscle fibres. In patients dying after the acute episode, the main pathological changes are seen in the heart valves which become thickened and distorted.

The arthritis has no specific pathological features. There is a non-specific infiltration of the synovium by inflammatory cells with some oedema. Rheumatic fever nodules are easily distinguished from rheumatoid nodules by their microscopic appearance, and are usually very much smaller to the naked eye.

Clinical Features

Rheumatic fever is rare in infants. The incidence increases in early childhood to reach a peak in the 5 to 15 year age group. Thereafter the incidence decreases quite sharply, although occasionally the disease may occur in young adults. The acute phase of rheumatic fever usually follows some three weeks after a sore throat, although some patients give no history of a throat infection. The onset is marked by the sudden development of a high temperature and an arthritis. The pyrexia is sustained, in contrast to the swinging fever of Still's disease (Fig. 11.2).

The arthritis is classically described as migratory, that is, it flits from joint to joint without leaving any damage. Many joints may be involved for short periods. On the other hand one or more joints may be the site of an acute synovitis for several weeks. The arthritis may involve one joint only, in which case aspiration and attempted culture of organisms from synovial fluid is required to differentiate it from septic arthritis. The synovial fluid is always sterile in rheumatic fever. There are several other features of rheumatic fever which may occur during the course of the disease. It would be very unusual for a single patient to show all these features, so it must be remembered that any combination of them—or none of them at all—may occur in addition to the acute attack. The most important effect of rheumatic fever is on the heart.

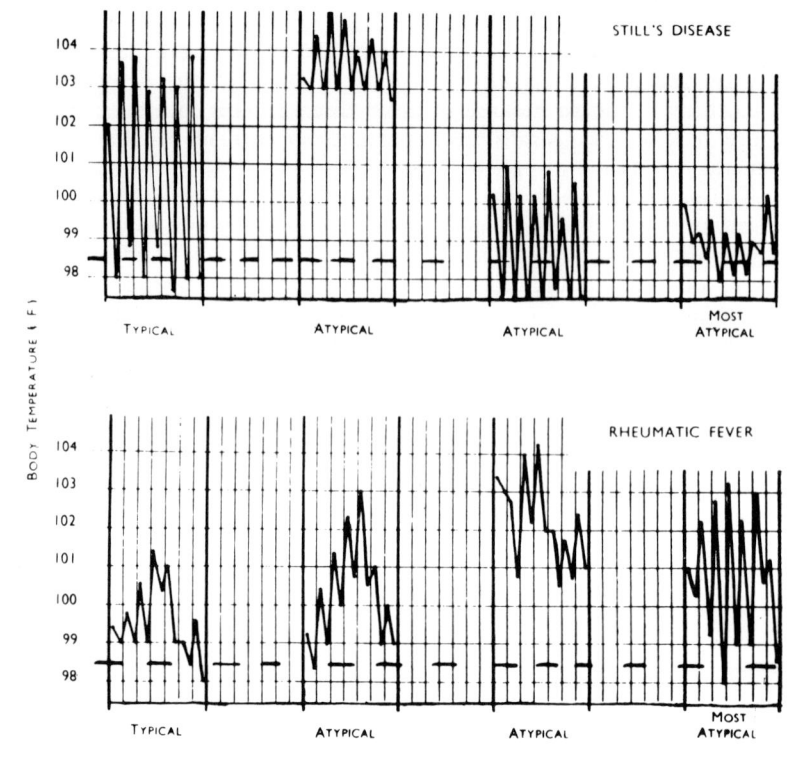

Fig. 11.2. The temperature charts of patients with rheumatic fever compared with Still's disease.

This may take many forms from a delay in conduction of the heart's electrical impulse seen on the electrocardiograph to gross cardiac failure leading to death. The important clinical signs are the development of murmurs heard with the stethoscope and enlargement of the heart detected clinically or by x-rays. If cardiac failure occurs this indicates a bad outlook. Chorea (St Vitus' Dance) is another manifestation of rheumatic fever. This condition is characterised by involuntary muscular spasms and emotional lability. The muscular movements are abrupt and purposeless usually involving the hands and face. The facial spasms give rise to bizarre grimaces which may involve the tongue as well as the facial muscles. The hand movements make the child clumsy and unable to perform tasks such as writing. The movements disappear during sleep. They cannot be controlled by the patient, and occur both at rest and during movement. The emotional lability is

Rheumatic Fever

characterised by sudden outbursts of crying or aggression. Examination may reveal weakness of the muscles and a 'pendular' knee jerk, i.e. when the knee jerk is tested the lower leg may swing backwards and forwards several times rather than once. Chorea occurs in girls more frequently than boys, and is commonest in the 10 to 15 year age group. It typically starts some months after the initial streptococcal infection. Occasionally the acute febrile phase is absent or unnoticed, but these patients remain at risk of developing rheumatic valvular disease in later life.

The skin may be affected in rheumatic fever by erythema marginatum, the presence of this rash being diagnostic of the disease. The rash occurs on the trunk or limbs. It starts with one or more central red patches. Each patch gradually expands, the centre returning to normal. The result is a series of irregular patches with red raised margins and, frequently pale centres. Other less characteristic rashes may occur, including erythema nodosum.

Rheumatic fever nodules are subcutaneous lumps varying in size from very small, barely palpable nodules to quite large swellings. They are firm and painless, and there are no signs of inflammation on the overlying skin. Their usual position is over bony prominences or tendon sheaths, and they vary from one to several dozen in number. The development of rheumatic fever nodules is usually a sign of severe disease, and they particularly occur where there is active carditis.

Investigations

As has been seen, the clinical signs of rheumatic fever may be very variable both in type and severity. Unfortunately laboratory tests are not very helpful in the diagnosis of this disease, though they are of assistance during its course. The presence of streptococcal infections can be detected by testing for antibodies against streptolysin. During the course of a streptococcal infection, the amount of this substance in the blood increases. This increase is detected by measuring the amount of antibody to it which the body produces. The amount of antibody is reported as the Anti-streptolysin O (ASO) titre. While a rising titre confirms the presence of an active infection, or a high titre suggests a recent infection with streptococci, this only proves the presence of the infection, not that the infection has caused rheumatic fever. More direct evidence of streptococcal infection may be obtained by culture of a throat swab. Absence of streptococci on the culture does not, however, mean that the disease is not rheumatic fever, as the initiating infection might have settled before the signs of rheumatic fever appear. The Erythrocyte Sedimentation Rate (ESR) gives a good guide to the severity of the inflammation taking place. However, any kind of inflammation or infection may cause a rise in the ESR so that it can be used as a guide to severity but not diagnosis. Electrocardiography may reveal the presence of abnormal conduction, or provide evidence of inflammatory disease in the heart, but does not reveal the cause of the disordered function it reveals. In summary, therefore, the laboratory can only be used to confirm clinical suspicion and help assess the severity of rheumatic fever. There is no diagnostic laboratory test.

Differential Diagnosis

Three of the most painful types of arthritis encountered are rheumatic fever, gout and pyogenic arthritis. Gout is distinguished by the fact that the big toe joint (1st metatarsophalangeal joint) is commonly involved, that the arthritis is not migratory, and there is a raised serum uric acid. Pyogenic arthritis usually affects only one joint, but if the diagnosis is considered the joint must be aspirated. The arthritis of rheumatic fever is migratory, usually affecting patients under 15 years of age. It is helped dramatically by full dosage salicylates. These points help to distinguish it from rheumatoid arthritis.

Treatment

There is no evidence that the treatment of the acute attack of rheumatic fever makes any difference to the development of serious long-term cardiac damage. It is, therefore, essentially symptomatic.

It is usual to treat the initiating streptococcal infection with penicillin although this makes no difference to the attack of acute rheumatism then in progress. It is of great importance to continue prophylactic antibiotic treatment on a long term basis. Patients who have had one attack of rheumatic fever are more susceptible than the general population to a second attack with the consequent risk of increasing any cardiac damage. Prophylaxis is usually continued until the patient is aged 20 or until five years after the initial attack whichever is the later. Either oral penicillin is given on a once or twice daily basis, or a long-acting penicillin (such as benzathine penicillin) is given monthly. The long acting preparation has the advantage of supervised dosage as it is given by intramuscular injection, but the process of injection is disliked by many patients, especially children. Sulphonamides may also be effective in prophylactic therapy, and the new long-acting preparations given on a once weekly basis may provide a convenient form of treatment.

During the acute attack it is customary for the patient to be put to bed. As with many paediatric conditions the traditional duration of bed rest is too long. The object of rest in bed was to reduce activity and thus reduce the work done by the heart. In fact, children in bed are sufficiently active for this difference in work to be negligible. Acutely inflamed joints obviously need rest, and may need splintage, especially of ankles, to keep them in good position. It is probably wise, despite the little objective evidence of reduced activity, to keep children with signs of active carditis in bed. The tradition of keeping the patient on bed rest until the ESR has fallen to normal does not seem to do the patient any good.

During the acute attack, the temperature may be reduced and the joint inflammation relieved by the use of salicylates. These should be given in full anti-inflammatory dosage, either by increasing the dose until tinnitus is produced and then maintaining the patient on a dose just below that which produced tinnitus, or by checking the plasma salicylate level and keeping this between 25 and 35 mg/100 ml. Salicylates may cause a dramatic effect in lowering the temperature and decreasing joint symptoms, but they have no effect on the all-important cardiac involvement. Corticosteroids have been advocated in the treatment of acute rheumatism. Their effect on the pyrexia and the joints is more rapid than that of aspirin, but there is a tendency for the disease to flare up when the dose is reduced. Advocates of corticosteroids claim that their use reduces the effects of cardiac involvement. There is no evidence that low doses of corticosteroids alter the prognosis, and the effects of high doses have not been adequately studied in a controlled fashion. The joint study by British and American workers on this topic failed to produce a clear answer because of the great variability in the course of the disease. High dose corticosteroids are, however, often used on an empirical basis in patients in whom the carditis is becoming uncontrollable by other means, and who are developing signs of cardiac failure.

When cardiac failure does occur in the acute phase the prognosis is grave, since it is within this group of patients that death occurs. Treatment is the same as for cardiac failure from other causes, i.e. digoxin and diuretics, with appropriate control of disturbed heart rhythm. There is no specific treatment for chorea, though these patients may require sedation and, rarely, psychotherapy.

Sequelae

The importance of rheumatic fever lies less in the acute attack, which is usually controllable, than in the long term problems produced by the disease. It has been likened to 'a dog which licks joints and bites hearts'. This descriptive phrase correctly emphasises the importance of the sequelae to acute rheumatism.

Although many patients with rheumatic fever tend to have aches and pains in their joints for years afterwards, few develop a long-standing arthritis as part of the disease. There is such a condition called Jaccoud's arthropathy, but it is very rare. It bears a superficial resemblance to rheumatoid arthritis, with marked ulnar deviation of the fingers but little joint swelling. The function in these hands is good. Erosive changes do not develop in the joints, and blood tests for rheumatoid factor are negative. In contrast, the cardiac manifestations may be progressive and eventually fatal. The incidence of permanent heart damage related to the signs during the acute attack of rheumatic fever is shown in Fig. 11.3.

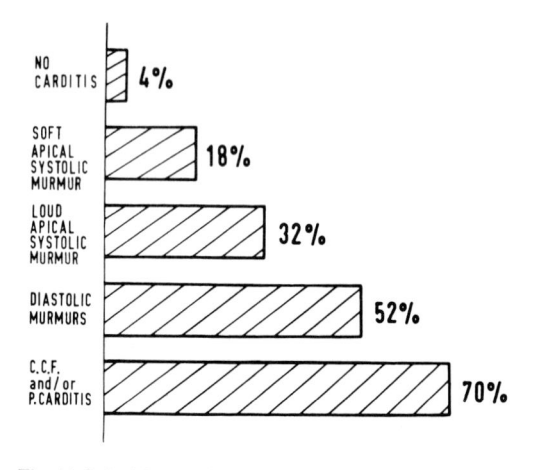

```
NO CARDITIS                    4%
SOFT APICAL SYSTOLIC MURMUR    18%
LOUD APICAL SYSTOLIC MURMUR    32%
DIASTOLIC MURMURS              52%
C.C.F. and/or P.CARDITIS       70%
```

Fig. 11.3. Incidence of heart disease five years after acute rheumatic fever related to the signs in the heart during the acute episode.

The long-term problems arise from disease of the heart valves which become thickened and deformed. In order of frequency the mitral, aortic and tricuspid valves are usually involved either alone or in combination. The disease may cause stenosis or incompetence of the valves, or a combination of these conditions. The development in surgical techniques has greatly improved the prognosis of patients with rheumatic heart disease, but valvular heart disease remains the major cause of disability and death caused by rheumatic fever.

12

Gout

Aetiology
Clinical Features
Investigations
Differential Diagnosis
Treatment
Conclusion

Gout is the rheumatic disease known for the longest time, and indeed until this century the majority of cases of arthritis were described as gout. True gout has influenced the course of history. It caused the Roman general Agrippa to commit suicide; it made Harvey, the discoverer of the circulation of blood, go out to dunk his gouty feet into iced water; it spurred George IV to invent long trousers to hide his swollen goaty feet; it soured the disposition of the great reformer, Martin Luther; it was instrumental in the loss of the American colonies in that Pitt who could have dealt with the crisis was prevented from going to the House of Commons because of an acute attack of gout; it caused Henry IV to postpone his marriage to Margaret of Anjou.

Aetiology

Gout is caused by accumulation of excess amounts of uric acid in the body. Uric acid is produced mainly from breakdown of the nucleic acids found in the nuclei of cells, and some uric acid is, therefore, found normally in the blood and urine. The channels of production and excretion of uric acid are shown in Fig. 12.1. The upper limit of normal blood uric acid is usually 0.40 m mol/l for women and 0.45 m mol/l for men. (The normal range in laboratories may vary because of different methods of measurement.) The distribution of levels is shown in Fig. 12.2. Excess uric acid may occur either where larger than normal amounts are produced or where excretion is poor. In clinical practice, however, gout is usually divided into primary and secondary.

Primary gout is that type of gout in which no obvious immediate cause of the high uric acid level can be found.

Secondary gout is that type in which there is an obvious immediate cause of the high uric acid level.

Some facts are known about the aetiology of primary gout. It is rarely found in pre-menopausal females or pre-pubertal males. The majority of cases (90%) are in young and middle-aged men, but the number of new cases in women after the menopause is the same as that

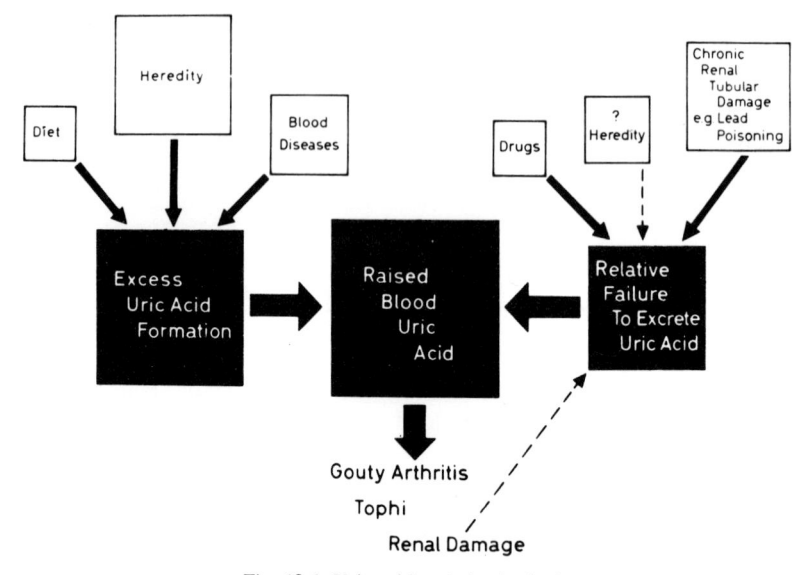

Fig. 12.1. Uric acid cycle in the body.

in men of the same age. In over a third there is a history of other members of the family being affected by gout. There is some evidence that gout is commoner in professional and managerial classes than in manual workers. Taking a diet high in purines found in foods such as sweetbreads and game, and alcohol, especially heavy wines, may increase the uric acid level.

Secondary gout occurs where there is a pathological increase in uric acid production or decrease in its excretion. As the main source of uric acid is cell nuclei, any condition in which there is an increased destruction of cells may lead to overproduction of uric acid. Blood diseases such as leukaemia may cause this because of the excess numbers of abnormal white blood cells being broken down. The treatment of malignant or non-malignant conditions by drugs, such as cytotoxic agents, which kill rapidly dividing cells, produces the same result. More commonly, secondary gout is caused by decreased excretion

Gout

of uric acid in the urine. This may happen as part of a general failure of the excretion mechanisms in the kidney, so that all forms of renal failure may cause high uric acid levels. A cause of increasing importance is the blocking of uric acid excretion by drugs. The commonest cause of this is the use of thiazide diuretics and frusemide, which prevent uric acid excretion by the kidney and hence cause its accumulation in the blood.

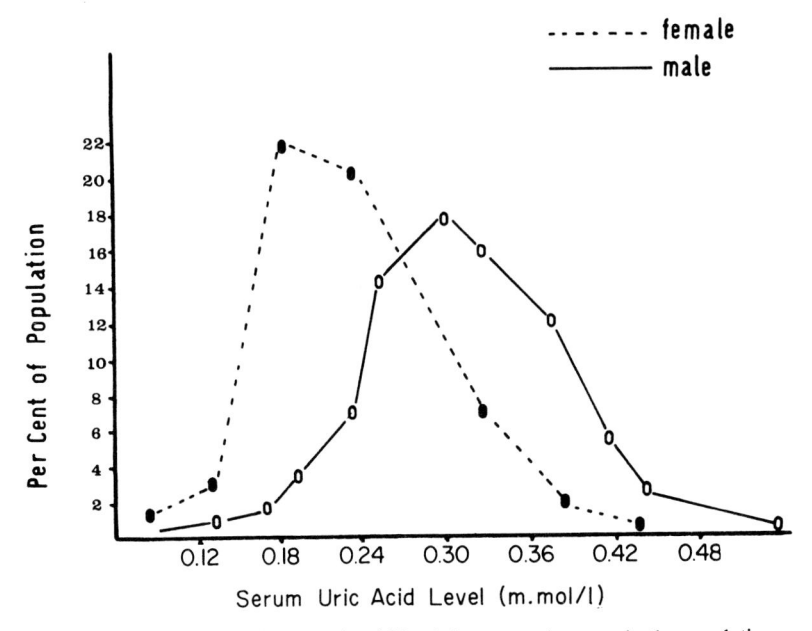

Fig. 12.2. Distribution of blood uric acid levels in men and women in the population.

All the conditions described above lead to high levels of uric acid in the blood, but not all patients with high plasma uric acid levels develop gout. The chances of suffering from gout increase as the plasma level of uric acid rises.

There is also a racial factor. Polynesian men have a high incidence of a raised serum uric acid in the blood (hyperuricaemia); it is present in over 40%. Similarly, there is a high incidence of gout.

Clinical Features

The characteristic clinical feature of gout is the occurrence of acute attacks of gouty arthritis. These comprise the sudden onset of excruciating pain in the affected joint, associated with redness and swelling. The joint is hot, and so exquisitely tender that the patient frequently cannot even bear the weight of the bedclothes on it. When Sidney Smith, the great wit, had an attack, he said: 'I feel as if I am walking on my eyeballs.' The metatarso-phalangeal joint of the big toe is the first to be affected in 76% of cases and remains the most commonly affected throughout the course of the disease (Fig. 12.3). Acute gout in the big toe is sometimes called by its old name 'podagra'.

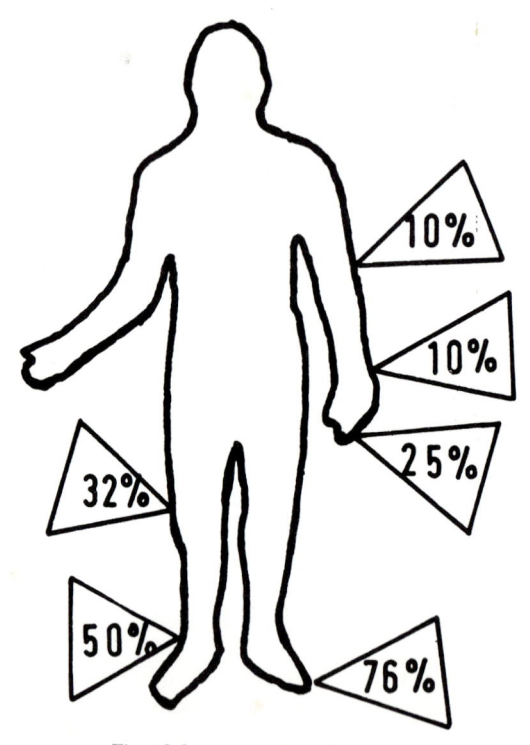

Fig. 12.3. Joint involved in gout.

Any other joint may be involved, the knee being next most frequent. If left untreated, the pain will remain agonising for some days. The joint will then slowly settle back to normal. As this occurs, the outer layers of the skin often peel from the area that was most severely inflamed. Once the joint has settled to normal there may be no signs of gout until a further attack occurs either in the same or another joint. This may occur after only a few weeks, or may be delayed for many years. Often there is some precipitating feature such as trauma. In hospital, acute

Gout

gout is frequently seen after an operation, as alterations in uric acid metabolism and excretion take place at the time of operation which make an acute attack more likely. A patient, therefore, being nursed on a surgical ward who develops an acute arthritis within two days of surgery is most likely to be suffering from gout. Another cause of gout is severely restricted calorie intake, amounting to starvation, for obesity over several weeks.

Although the dramatic nature of the acute attacks attracts the attention of both the patient and his attendants, greater damage may occur during the intervals between attacks. The acute attack is caused by the production of sodium urate crystals in the joint (Fig. 12.4). These are engulfed by white cells which rupture and release damaging

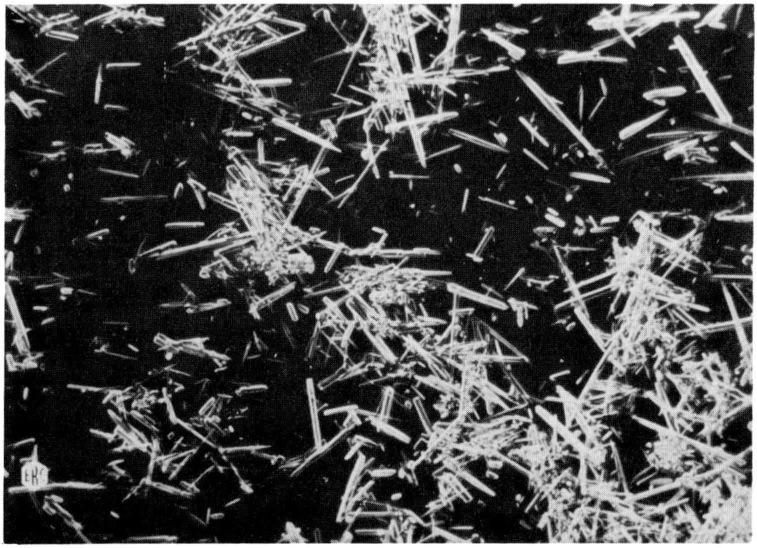

Fig. 12.4. Uric acid crystals.

enzymes. These cause the acute synovitis which is so characteristic of acute gout. Uric acid may, however, eventually become deposited in the joint causing erosion of the bone ends (Fig. 12.5). In contrast to rheumatoid arthritis, these erosions give the appearance of punched out holes in normal bone. A more obvious appearance of uric acid deposition is the formation of tophi. These are yellowish nodules which tend to occur especially over cartilage, particularly in the ear (Fig. 12.6). Before modern treatment was available, large tophi could spread to involve wide areas of the limbs. They would then tend to ulcerate, the

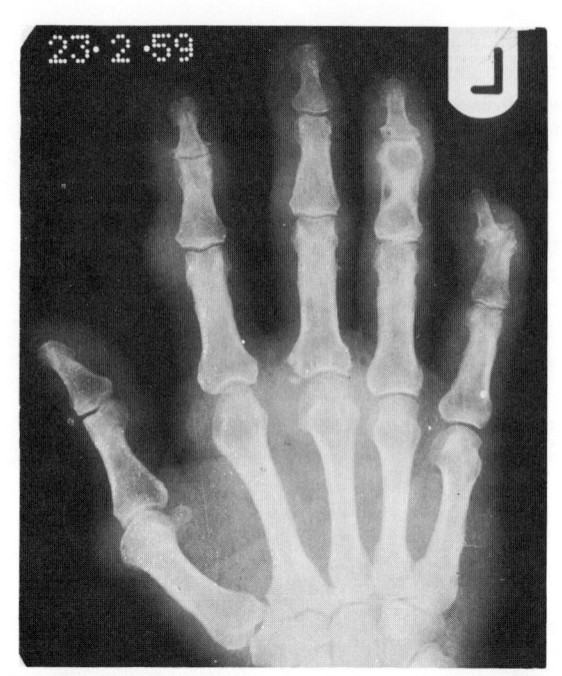

Fig. 12.5a. Urate deposits in the soft tissue giving a tophus around the proximal joint of the index fingers and in middle phalanx of the ring finger producing cysts.

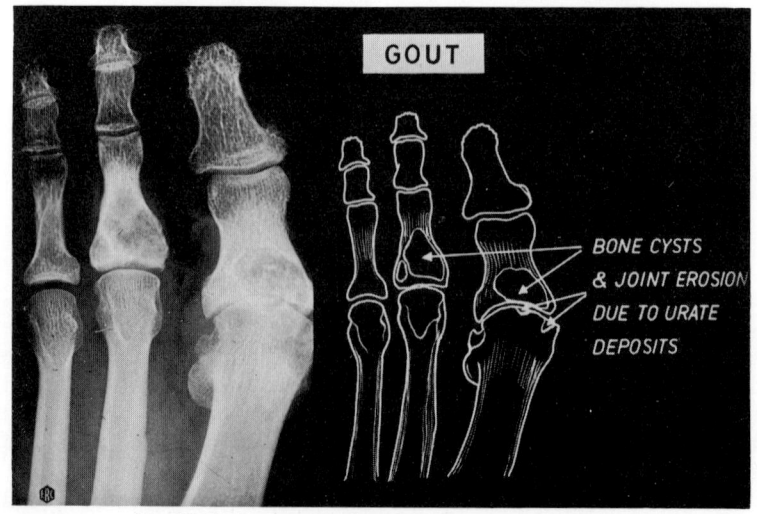

Fig. 12.5b. Tophaceous deposits in the bones of the toes.

uric acid being extruded from them. Of more clinical importance is the hidden deposition of uric acid in the kidneys. This can eventually lead to renal failure, and is potentially life-threatening.

The clinical course of gout, whether primary or secondary is, therefore, the appearance of acute attacks of gouty arthritis at variable intervals, with the possibility of uric acid deposition continuing unnoticed in the intervals.

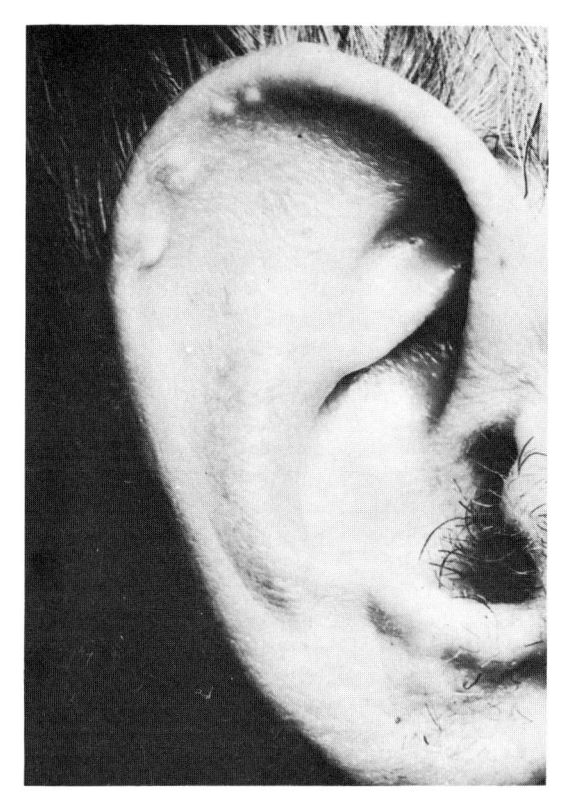

Fig. 12.6. Tophus in the ear.

Investigations

As well as a raised serum uric acid during an acute attack the erythrocyte sedimentation rate may be raised and the white blood count increased. There may be findings of other diseases that have produced secondary gout e.g. an increased haemoglobin concentration in polycythaemia or an increased white count with abnormal cells in leukaemia. Aspiration of joint fluid may reveal typical crystals in the fluid and this is the only absolute diagnostic test for gout. Deposition of uric acid in the bone and joints may produce characteristic x-ray lesions.

Differential Diagnosis

The three most painful arthritic conditions are gout, an infected joint (pyogenic arthritis) and rheumatic fever. Aspiration of the joint is mandatory to exclude a possible pyogenic arthritis. The migratory nature of the arthritis, and its occurrence some three weeks after a streptococcal sore throat will help to differentiate rheumatic fever. A gouty big toe is commonly misdiagnosed as cellulitis, and is frequently treated with antibiotics, or even lanced. Neither of these measures is beneficial and may aggravate the condition.

Attention has been directed recently to a condition called 'pseudo-gout'. This is also due to crystals in the joint, but this time they are of calcium pyrophosphate. It is diagnosed by finding calcification in fibrocartilage, especially of the knee, and by the finding of characteristic crystals in joint aspirate. The serum uric acid in this condition is usually normal but it may be associated with true gout.

Treatment

The treatment of acute gout is aimed at relieving the severe pain as rapidly as possible. The earlier in the course of the acute attack that treatment is started, the easier it is to abort. It is important, therefore, that patients at home are given a supply of tablets and instructions so that they can begin treatment as soon as the attack starts. The traditional remedy is colchicine 0.5 mg given two hourly for a maximum of 24 hours until the pain subsides or diarrhoea or vomiting occurs. This treatment has now been superceded by the use of phenylbutazone or indomethacin. The most effective regime appears to be indomethacin in the following dosage scheme:

    100 mg 4 hourly until most pain gone
 then 100 mg 8 hourly for 24 hours
 then   75 mg 8 hourly for 24 hours
 then   50 mg 8 hourly for 3 days.

Despite the high dose of indomethacin, side effects are unusual. Alternatively, phenylbutazone may be given in high doses (up to 200 mg 4 times daily by intramuscular injection for two days followed by 100 mg orally three times the next day). It is important that patients taking long term treatment for their gout continue their chronic medication *unchanged* throughout treatment of an acute attack.

In considering long term medication to reduce uric acid levels in the blood, the first decision to be made is whether or not such treatment is necessary. Once started, the therapy will be life-long. The decision to start treatment is influenced by high levels of uric acid in the blood, frequent acute attacks, the presence of gouty tophi and evidence of renal disease. If treatment is initiated, two possible ways of reducing the uric acid level are available. The traditional method is to give uricosuric agents, that is drugs which increase the excretion of uric acid in the urine. The main drug in this group is probenecid. This drug has been used over many years, and its few side effects are well known. The main disadvantage is that the amount of uric acid passed through the kidneys is increased, with the theoretical possibility that uric acid deposition there may also be increased. Other drugs have a uricosuric action. Sulphinpyrozone, a phenylbutazone derivative, is quite a powerful uricosuric agent, but is less popular in Britain than in continental Europe. Phenylbutazone itself has a uricosuric action in high dosage, but is never used alone for this purpose. It is important to remember that when phenylbutazone is used in the treatment of acute gout it is for its analgesic/anti-inflammatory properties, *not* as a uricosuric agent. The effect of aspirin on uric acid is very important. In low doses, below 4 g per day, it causes retention of uric acid. In doses above this level, it enhances uric acid excretion. As few patients take aspirin in doses greater than 4 g (13-14 tablets) daily, it is usual to advise patients with gout which is untreated or being treated with uricosuric agents not to take aspirin at any time. This is particularly so as it antagonises the effect of probenecid and sulphinpyrazone (Fig. 12.7). Phenylbutazone in low dose will also cause uric acid retention.

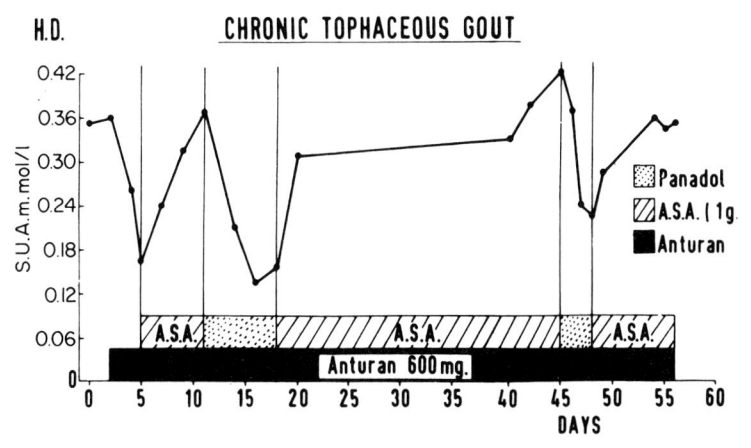

Fig. 12.7. The effect on the serum uric acid level of giving anturan (sulphinpyrazone) with aspirin which is antagonistic and with panadol which is not.

More recently a second method of reducing the plasma level of uric acid has been introduced. Allopurinol is a drug which interferes with the formation of uric acid by interfering with the enzyme xanthine oxidase which is essential in the pathway of formation of uric acid. This means that the amount of uric acid in the blood is reduced, as is the amount going through the kidneys. The body excretes substances which are precursors of uric acid, such as xanthine, all of which are more soluble than uric acid and therefore more easily excreted in the urine. Allopurinol is slowly replacing the uricosuric agents in many places, and increased experience with it suggests that it is a safe drug in long-term use. It is now the treatment of choice for patients with secondary gout, with tophi, or with very high plasma levels of uric acid. In other patients its advantages are weighed against the greater experience with uricosuric drugs. It may also be used prophylactically in situations where a sudden increase in serum uric acid is anticipated, as in the treatment of leukaemia with cytotoxic agents.

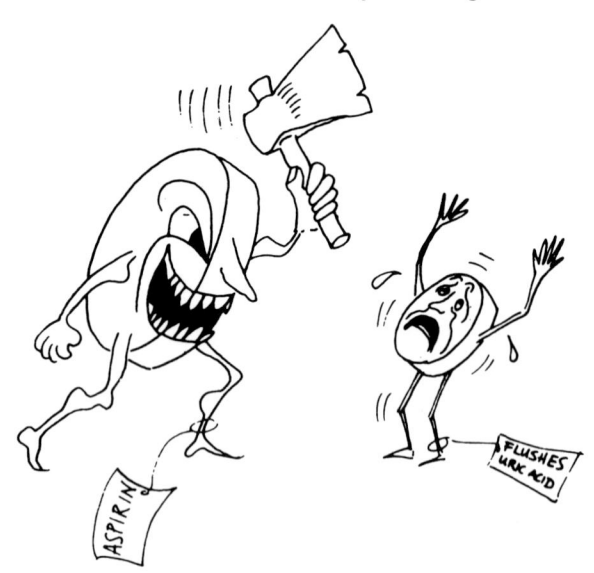

Aspirin has the effect of counteracting the action of these drugs.

Fig. 12.8. Picture from Gout Handbook (drawn by Dr John Moll).

When long term treatment is introduced the patient must be warned that an acute attack of gout may take place during the early weeks of therapy. In order to reduce the chance of such an acute attack taking place it is usual to add a small dose of colchicine (0.5 mg twice daily) for the first 3-6 months of long term therapy. Acute attacks occurring at any time while on long term treatment are treated as outlined previously, with continuation of the long term regime unchanged.

From the nursing point of view a cradle may need to be arranged over an acute gouty joint to prevent the weight of the bedclothes aggravating the pain. In hot weather gouty patients should be encouraged to take extra fluid to prevent the concentration of urate crystals in the kidneys.

Diet is not thought to be such an important factor with the advent of effective drugs to control the uric acid level, but nevertheless, the sufferer should be advised to moderate his alcoholic intake and to refrain from high purine foods. An excellent booklet written for patients with gout is produced by the Arthritis and Rheumatism Council. In our studies at Leeds of doctor-patient communication we have found that it is much appreciated by patients. In further investigations we are evaluating a completely illustrated book (drawn by Dr John Moll)—an example of the illustrations is shown in Fig. 12.8. This illustrated booklet is not yet generally available.

Surgery is known to provoke acute attacks, and immediate treatment should be available if needed after an operation. Before the advent of long term treatment, gross tophi were sometimes removed surgically, and this may still be done to hasten the resolution of the uric acid pool.

Conclusion

Gout has been described many times in past centuries, and certain of its mysteries remain unsolved. It is, however, one of the few rheumatic diseases for which treatment exists that can eliminate almost all its discomforts and dangers.

13
Disorders of the Foot

Foot Disorders as Part of a General Disease
  Rheumatoid arthritis
  Osteoarthrosis
  Ankylosing spondylitis
  Gout
  Psoriatic arthritis
  Treatment
Local Disorders of the Foot
  Disorders of the forefoot
    Hallux valgus
    Hallux rigidus
    Hammer toe
    Metatarsalgia
  Disorders of the arches of the foot
    Flat feet
    Pes cavus
  Disorders of the hindfoot
    Plantar fasciitis
    Achilles tendinitis

Transmission of the entire weight of the body to the ground takes place through the feet. They are also subject to trauma from the ground, from the person standing on them, from their footwear and also from things being dropped on them. It is, therefore, not surprising that both major and minor disorders of the foot are common in rheumatological and orthopaedic practice.

In general, the congenital disorders of the foot are the province of the orthopaedic surgeon, and will not be further considered. Similarly tumours affecting the bones of the foot fall in the province of surgery. Both rheumatological and orthopaedic units however, see patients with a wide spectrum of foot disorders. These can conveniently be considered under two headings:
    1. Foot disorders as part of a general disease
    2. Local disorders of the foot.

Before considering individual conditions some general points about examination of the foot must be considered. Feet are designed for standing, and it is essential that both the weightbearing surface, the sole, and the processes of weightbearing and walking must be considered. Footwear can be either beneficial or detrimental to the feet, high fashion usually being harmful. The patient's shoes must be examined at the same time as the patient and note taken not only of the style and fit of the shoes but the pattern of wear on the soles and heels.

Foot Disorders as Part of a General Disease

All the various types of polyarthritis may affect the foot. The relationships of the various bones of the feet are shown in Fig. 13.1.

Rheumatoid arthritis

This may affect any or all of the foot joints, but the burden of the disease usually falls on the metatarso-phalangeal joints. These often become subluxed, and painful; tender metatarsal heads can often be seen on looking at the sole of the foot.

Flexion of the subluxed toes causes the interphalangeal joint to press against the inside of the shoe producing at least corns and often chronically abraded and infected areas. Rheumatoid involvement of the midtarsal and subtaloid joints should be carefully defined by examination, as local corticosteroid injections into these joints—a difficult procedure—often produces considerable benefit. It must be remembered that these are weightbearing joints and that rest after injection is important. Subtaloid and hindfoot joint disease is often loosely called 'ankle disease', but it is the addition of arthritis in these joints to disease in the ankle joints which may produce inversion or eversion of the foot and considerably increase the amount of pain produced.

The hands and feet tend to be the parts of the body involved first in rheumatoid arthritis. It is always useful to x-ray the feet, even if they are asymptomatic, where the diagnosis is in doubt, as erosive changes may be seen early in the course of the disease. Of 1,953 new cases of rheumatoid arthritis at Leeds 19% had the feet predominantly involved and in 37% the feet and other joints were involved.

Osteoarthrosis

Radiological changes of osteoarthrosis may be seen as part of generalised osteoarthrosis, but more problems usually arise from localised disease.

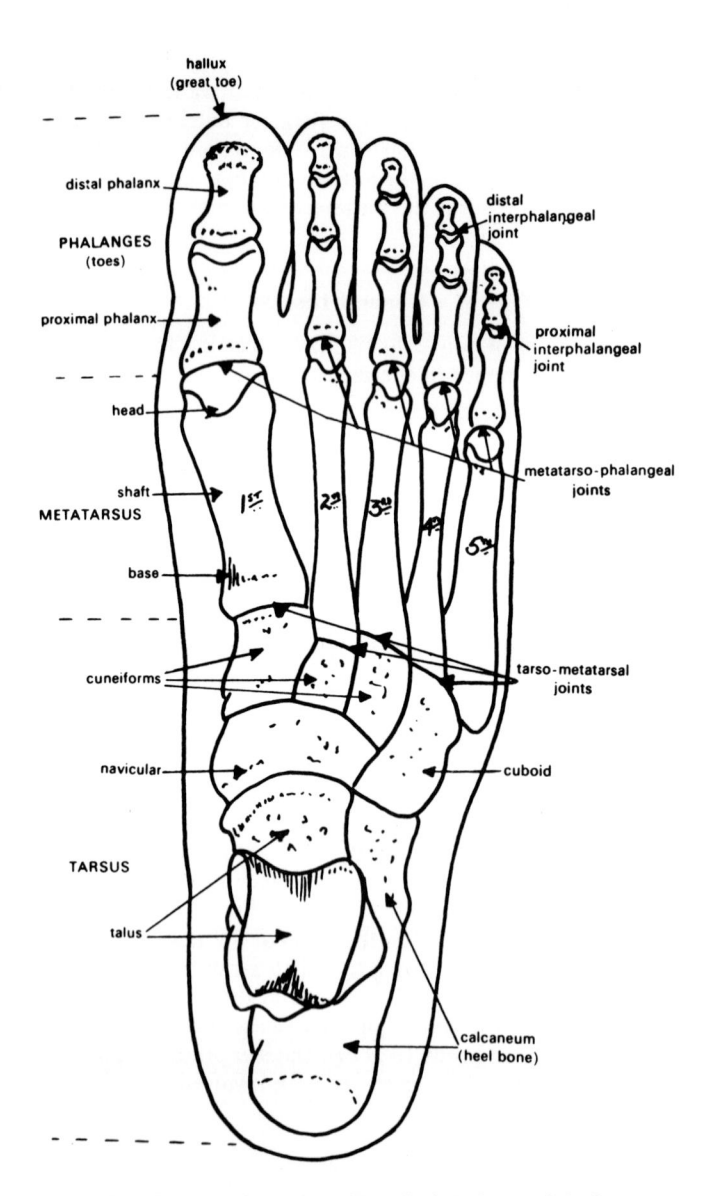

Fig. 13.1. View from above (dorsal) of the bones of the foot.

Ankylosing spondylitis

This may affect the foot, not only because of involvement of the joints but also because of such conditions as plantar fasciitis and Achilles tendinitis which may be associated with it. These conditions are considered later.

Gout

Gout frequently affects the feet, the first metatarso-phalangeal joints being the most common site of acute attacks. The agony may be excruciating.

Psoriatic arthritis

Involvement of the feet in psoriatic arthritis is similar to that in the hands. A striking association between nail and joint changes in the same toe may be seen, and 'sausage toes' may be produced like 'sausage fingers' by tendon sheath as well as joint involvement.

Treatment

The treatment of these conditions when they affect the feet is usually the control of the general disease. Surgery may be helpful in the correction of metatarsalgia; though triple arthrodesis of the hindfoot is often unsuccessful in rheumatoid patients. Removal of the toes, called the Pobble operation after Edward Lear's *The Pobble who lost his toes* sounds horrifying but is greatly appreciated by patients who have toes which are useless, deformed, painful appendages. Simpler measures include the provision of chiropody, which is required by 50% of patients attending rheumatology clinics, and of made-to-measure shoes, which we have shown to be among the most valuable of appliances supplied to patients.

Local Disorders of the Foot

These can be conveniently considered in three groups:
1. Disorders of the forefoot,
2. Disorders of the arches of the foot,
3. Disorders of the hindfoot.

Disorders of the forefoot

These are very common and particularly involve the great toe.

Hallux valgus is the deviation of the great toe away from the midline. This causes pressure on the adjacent toes, the great toe eventually taking up a position crossed above or below them. The first metatarso-phalangeal joint shows bony enlargement which is usually, though not invariably, covered by a bursa called a bunion. This may be the site of severe inflammation and pain, often chronic and occasionally associated with infection. Tight fitting shoes and socks or stockings frequently predispose to this condition (Fig. 13.2). Treatment in the early stage may require only the separation of the first and second toes by a shaped foam pad. Later cases are usually treated by surgery (Fig. 13.3).

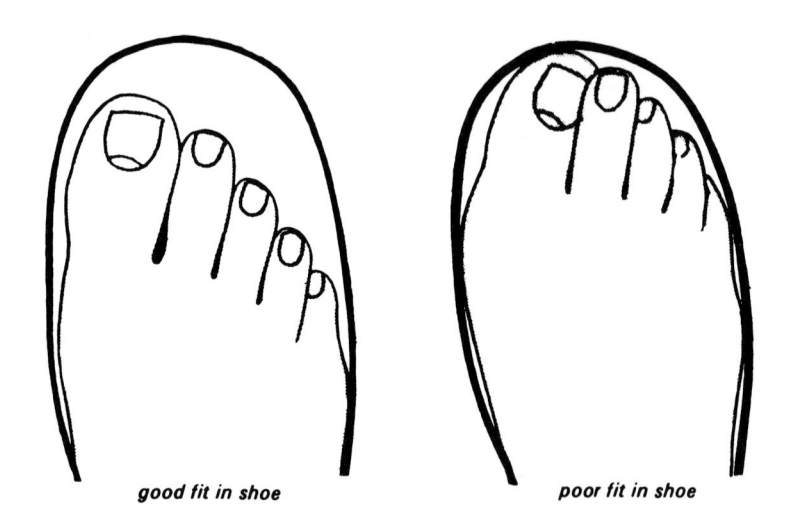

good fit in shoe   *poor fit in shoe*

Fig. 13.2. The importance of a good fitting shoe.

Hallux rigidus causes loss of movement at the metatarso-phalangeal joint of the great toe. Severe osteoarthrotic changes are seen in this joint on x-ray, with narrowing of the joint space, sclerosis of the bony margin and osteophyte formation. The symptoms of mild cases may be relieved by appropriate soft padding or by a bar under the sole of the shoe, but severe cases require surgery.

Hammer toe (Fig. 13.4) usually occurs in the second and third toe. The toe is bent up in an inverted V shape to give a high knuckle. This defect may be congenital, or it may begin in childhood, usually caused by pressure from a short narrow shoe or a short tight sock. A callus usually develops on the prominent part of the toe which rubs against

Disorders of the Foot

the shoe. This results in pain. A similar condition may complicate rheumatoid arthritis, when the metatarso-phalangeal joint has subluxated.

Appropriate footwear may help to relieve the pressure and pain. Surgically, arthroplasty may be done. A small part of the bone is removed to let a fibrous joint form. The toe is splinted into the new shape.

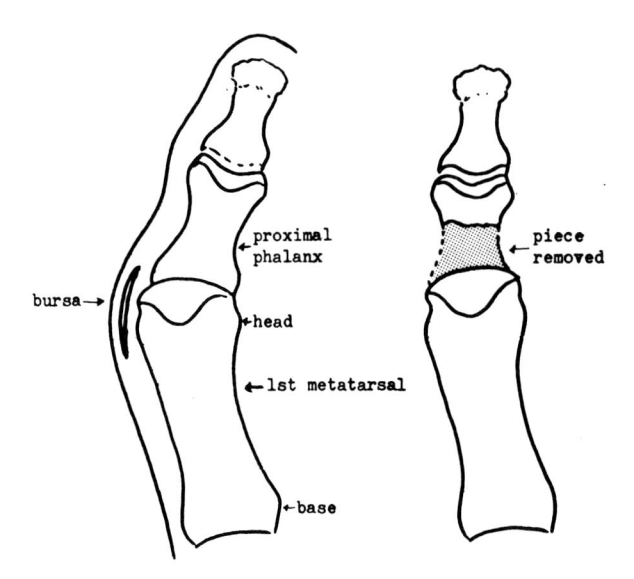

Fig. 13.3. Hallux valgus and a Keller's operation to rectify it.

Metatarsalgia is the production of pain under the metatarsal heads without obvious pathological cause. Although high arches or inappropriate footwear may be found, there is often no obvious precipitating cause. Sometimes it is the first sign of rheumatoid arthritis. The pain may be intense and prevent walking. Callus formation may be seen on the sole of the foot. Treatment is either by use of an appropriate soft insole or an external 'metatarsal bar' fitted to the shoes.

Disorders of the arches of the foot

The most common disorder in this area is *flat feet*. In these the natural antero-posterior arch of the foot is lost and the patient stands with the feet abducted. The flat foot may appear normal on non-weightbearing examination, but standing reveals the abnormal position. Although many patients complain of pain of varying severity in the feet, others complain simply of 'tired' feet, while some present with muscular pains in the lower leg caused by the abnormal posture. Treatment is firstly by encouraging the use of properly fitting shoes, as poor footwear is the commonest precipitating cause. Foot exercises are usually beneficial, though some patients will require the provision of appropriate arch supports.

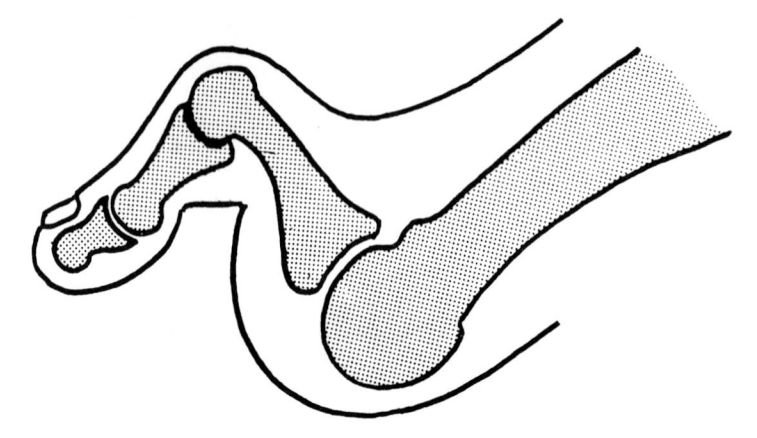

Fig. 13.4. Hammer toe.

Pes cavus. The opposite to flat foot is the high arch of pes cavus (Fig. 13.5). In its more extreme form this is usually the result of a congenital abnormality or a neurological disorder such as poliomyelitis. Patients with symptoms from arches which are at the 'high' end of the normal range should wear arch supports. The management of this and other minor foot conditions is well discussed in a book by the Consumers' Association, *Care of the Feet.*

Disorders of the hindfoot

The insertion of the plantar fascia into the calcaneum (os calcis) is the site of the pain of *plantar fasciitis.* This may be associated with ankylosing spondylitis or Reiter's disease but is often a solitary occurrence. The site of the insertion is painful on weightbearing and the pain may be reproduced during examination by local pressure. X-ray may show a plantar spur, but this may be irrelevant as these are seen about as frequently in normal people. The pain may be relieved by

pes cavus

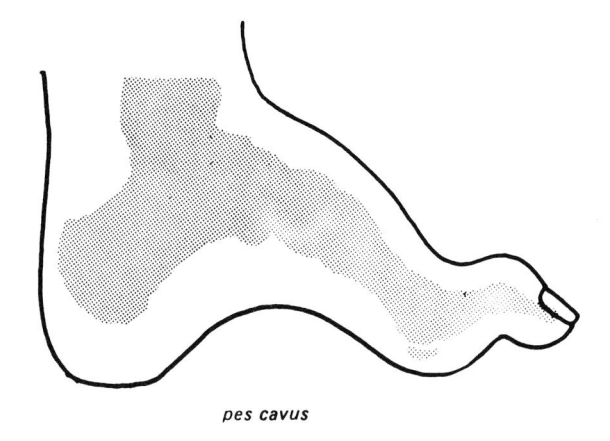

impression of foot

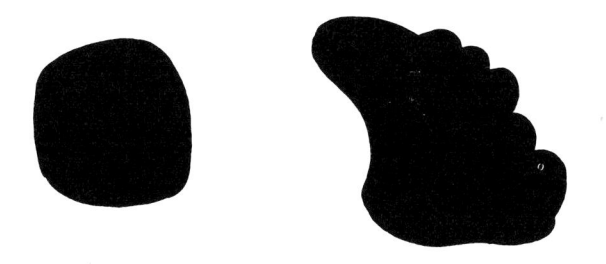

Fig. 13.5. Pes cavus.

wearing a soft rubber pad in the shoe, but local injection of hydrocortisone and local anaesthetic may be needed. This is usually effective but is, although brief, a painful process during which the patient will require a high degree of encouragement and comfort from the nurse.

Achilles tendinitis may also occur as a part of generalised disease but is often seen alone. The tender, swollen tendon sheath is easily identified. It may have been produced or exacerbated by a rigid, tight shoe heel, and responds to relief of pressure, rest and corticosteroid injection if necessary. Rupture of the Achilles tendon may be a dramatic event, but *central core degeneration* has recently been recognised as a condition causing pain and swelling in the Achilles tendon as a result of overuse,

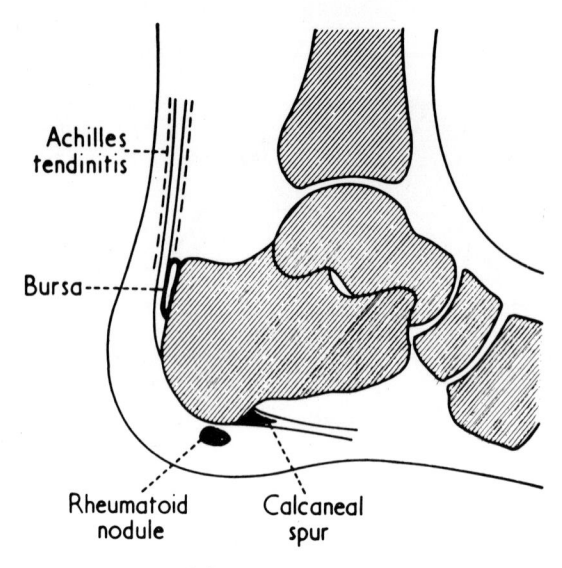

Fig. 13.6. Disorders around the heel.

especially in athletes. Surgical excision of the diseased centre of the tendon may be required. Various changes which may occur around the heel are shown in Fig. 13.6 and these include an Achilles tendinitis, Achilles or calcanean bursitis, a rheumatoid nodule under the heel, or plantar fasciitis with or without a calcanean spur.

14
Miscellaneous Types of Arthritis

Psoriatic Arthritis
Distal type
Identical type
Deforming type
Prognosis
Treatment
Arthritis and Bowel Disease
Enteropathic arthritis
Ankylosing spondylitis
Whipple's disease
Hypertrophic Pulmonary Osteoarthropathy
Polymyalgia Rheumatica

A number of conditions have not fallen into the categories discussed elsewhere. These are collected here for convenience, not necessarily because any association exists between them.

Psoriatic Arthritis

For many years it was considered that patients with psoriasis were unusually liable to develop rheumatoid arthritis. Careful studies have shown that this is not so. Psoriatic patients are neither more nor less liable than the general population to develop true rheumatoid disease. They may, however, develop a similar, but separate condition called 'psoriatic arthritis'. This condition exists in three forms—distal, identical and deforming. Each type may be complicated by the presence of sacro-iliitis with or without clinical ankylosing spondylitis.

A number of famous people have been afflicted by this disease. The actress who plays Mrs Dale in Mrs Dale's Diary on the BBC described her case in the magazine of the British Rheumatism Association. The case of Dennis Potter, author of the controversial play 'Son of Man' was also vividly described in the *Daily Telegraph Magazine* on April 2nd, 1969.

'Dennis Potter might be the survivor of some grim inquisition. His

135

painful limp a legacy of the boot. His fingers twisted and the nails blunted an opaque yellow by screwed instruments. In fact, he has been crippled on and off for 7 of his 35 years. He suffers from arthritis and also psoriasis, the malevolent skin condition which seems to have no organic cause except—in certain cases—a primitive link with the cycle of the year, abating in the summer sunlight only to return with the first dark days of winter . . . sometimes he blames the bomb, the wrongness of the world; at other times he dates it all back to the onset of guilt he felt when as a Forest of Dean miner's son who had been to Oxford he returned home with a TV unit to make a patronising documentary about his part of the world, his village, his family . . . but Potter himself is back in bed with a regression of the illness. His face and arms are aflame. He winces as his joints scrape and click. He sips milk laced with whisky and chain-smokes Players Gold Leaf. When the illness is at its worst he cannot even eat, for his jaw muscles seize; he cannot read for the psoriasis gums up his eyelids . . . I wrote most of the play in six weeks in hospital in Birmingham . . . the pen had to be strapped to my hand because I could not hold it. The paper got sploshed with the steroid grease they were putting on my skin.'

Patients with psoriasis frequently have a family history of the condition. Extensive family studies in our unit have shown that the relatives of patients with psoriatic arthritis are more likely than their wives or the general population to have psoriasis, psoriatic arthritis, sacro-iliitis, ankylosing spondylitis and ulcerative colitis.

Distal type

Distal psoriatic arthritis is the classical form of the disease. The nails are involved by psoriasis, and the adjacent distal interphalangeal joints develop an inflammatory arthritis. This may sometimes be 'topographical' in that either the nail and the joint are involved or both are spared. This disease is distinguished from primary generalised osteo-arthrosis, which also affects the distal joints, by the inflammatory rather than bony swelling, the presence of erosions rather than osteophytes on x-rays (Fig. 14.1), and the nail involvement by psoriasis. While the nails may be severely deformed by the disease, at other times the only sign of psoriasis is the presence of small pits in the nail (Fig. 14.2). The disease may spread to involve other joints in the fingers and toes, and less commonly, elsewhere.

Identical type

The identical type of psoriatic arthritis is so called because of its resemblance to true rheumatoid arthritis. There are, however, several

Miscellaneous Types of Arthritis 137

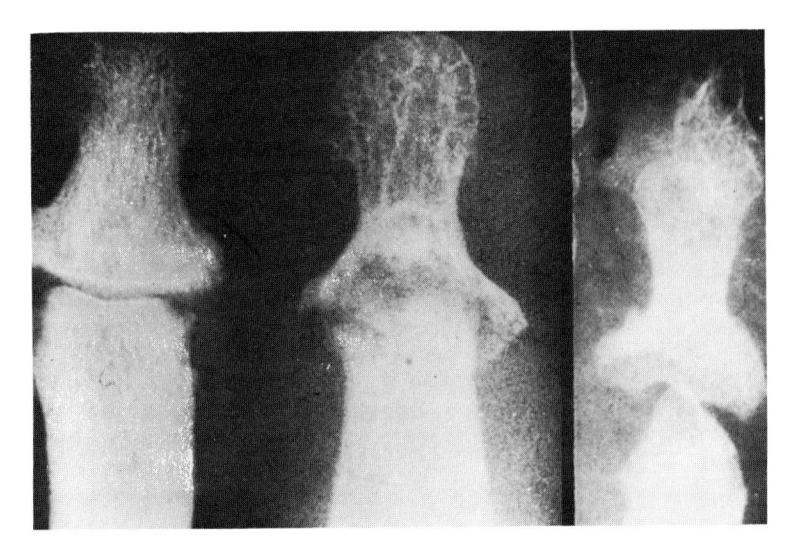

Fig. 14.1. Progressive changes in the distal interphalangeal joint of a patient with psoriatic arthritis.

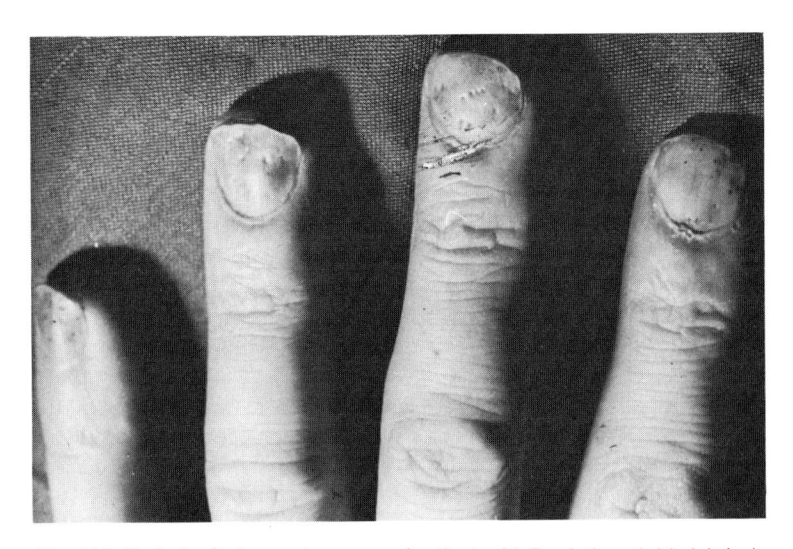

Fig. 14.2. Typical nail changes in a group of patients with Psoriatic arthritis (pitting).

distinguishing features. The polyarthritis of rheumatoid disease is usually symmetrical when fully developed, whereas the psoriatic pattern is more patchy. Rheumatoid nodules are not formed in psoriatic arthritis, and no rheumatoid factor is found in the blood. Finally, patients with psoriasis are prone to develop 'sausage fingers'. These get their name from the diffuse swelling of the affected finger, which contrasts with the more usual spindle-shaped swelling of rheumatoid arthritis. Spindle-shaped swelling is produced by inflammation in the proximal interphalangeal joint, with relative normality elsewhere, whereas the sausage finger is the site of synovitis in both the flexor and extensor tendons, giving rise to the more diffuse swelling. In contrast to rheumatoid arthritis there are few extra-articular manifestations of the disease. No severe systemic upsets such as neuropathy, vasculitis or lung changes occur but inflammation of the eye may be present.

Deforming type

As in rheumatoid arthritis, a small number of patients may go on to develop a severe destructive arthritis. This produces 'opera glass' fingers and toes, so called because the digit can be pulled in and out like an opera glass. These patients often have sacro-iliitis as well. Sacro-iliac changes may, however, occur in the other forms of the disease, and full-blown ankylosing spondylitis may develop. It is suggested that x-rays of patients with the psoriatic form of spondylitis are more liable to show large areas of calcification in the ligaments around the spine, although this appearance is not specific to psoriatics.

Prognosis

In general the outlook for patients with psoriatic arthritis is better than that of rheumatoid arthritis. Many patients experience a flare-up of their arthritis when their skin is bad, the arthritis resolving as the skin improves. Others feel that their skin and joint problems alternate and some may show no relationship between the two.

Treatment

The treatment of psoriatic arthritis is similar to that of rheumatoid arthritis. However, anti-malarial drugs (e.g., chloroquine) should not be used, as they may increase the severity of the skin disease. Gold may be used, since a drug rash does not occur any more frequently nor is the psoriasis aggravated. Corticosteroids are used less frequently than in rheumatoid arthritis. Great care must be taken with injections into joints if these are adjacent to skin lesions, since psoriatic plaques harbour bacteria. Surgical incisions through the skin do not take longer to heal than normal.

Arthritis and Bowel Disease

Enteropathic arthritis

The inflammatory gut diseases, ulcerative colitis and Crohn's disease, may be associated with arthritis of two types. The first is called 'enteropathic arthritis' which is an inflammatory synovitis involving large and lower limb joints more than small and upper limb ones. The knee is the most commonly involved joint (Figs. 14.3 and 14.4). It occurs at the time of presentation or during the course of the intestinal disease, and tends to occur where the disease is extensive or accompanied by other complications such as perianal sepsis. This arthritis is self limiting, and patients can be reassured that they will not be crippled by the arthritis. X-rays do not show joint damage. If the gut disease is cured, for example by procto-colectomy in ulcerative colitis, the joint disease does not recur.

Ankylosing spondylitis

The second type of arthritis is ankylosing spondylitis. Whereas enteropathic arthritis appears to be caused by something in the gut, and can be considered as a 'side effect' of gut disease, ankylosing spondylitis is found because there is an hereditary tendency to develop both diseases. They are, however, completely independent; that is, the course and treatment of one disease does not affect the other. Sacro-iliitis may be seen on x-rays, such as barium studies, taken for the gut disease, and should serve as a warning sign.

Whipple's disease

This is a very rare gut disease in which characteristic cells are found in the small intestine when a biopsy is taken. Arthritis similar to that found in colitis occurs in nearly all patients with Whipple's disease, and is the first sign of the disease in 60%.

Hypertrophic Pulmonary Osteoarthropathy

Finger clubbing is seen in many conditions, particularly cyanotic congenital heart disease, bronchiectasis, inflammatory gut disease and

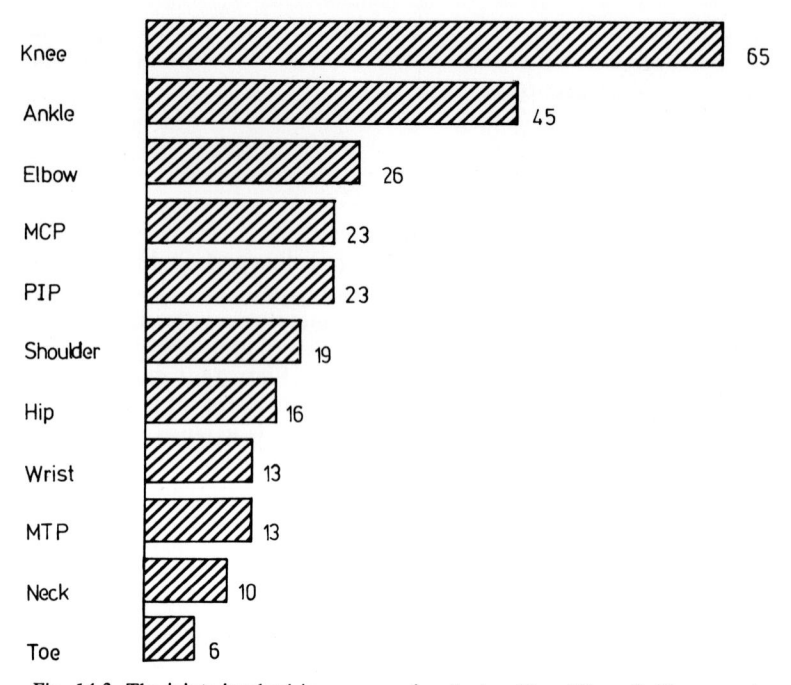

Joint	Count
Knee	65
Ankle	45
Elbow	26
MCP	23
PIP	23
Shoulder	19
Hip	16
Wrist	13
MTP	13
Neck	10
Toe	6

Fig. 14.3. The joints involved in a group of patients with colitic arthritis, seen at Leeds.

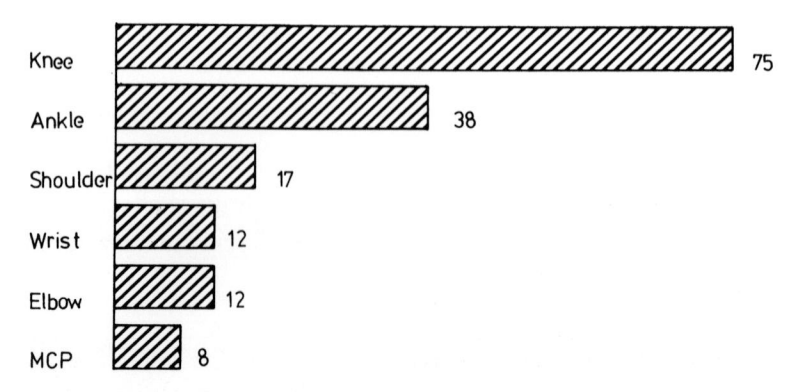

Joint	Count
Knee	75
Ankle	38
Shoulder	17
Wrist	12
Elbow	12
MCP	8

Fig. 14.4. The joints involved in a group of patients with the arthritis of Crohn's disease, seen at Leeds.

carcinoma of lung. Associated with this some patients develop acute inflammation of the wrists and ankles. This is due to inflammation of the periosteum of the long bones of the forearm and legs near the joints. Occasionally swelling of the knees occurs as part of hypertrophic pulmonary osteoarthropathy. A striking example is shown in Figs. 14.5-14.7. In this case the patient was a dog with a mesothelioma of the pleura.

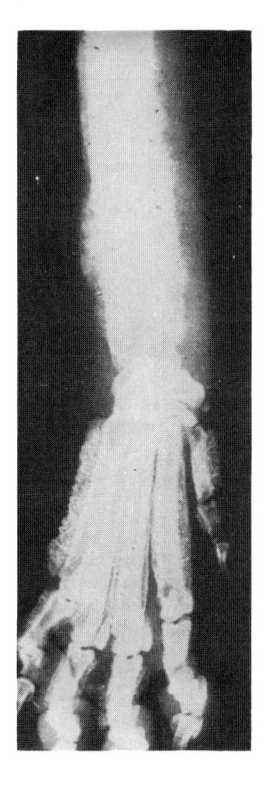

Fig. 14.5. Periosteal reaction in a patient with hypertrophic pulmonary osteoarthropathy.

Polymyalgia Rheumatica

This is usually found in patients aged 55 or over. Women are more frequently affected. The characteristic symptoms are pain and severe morning stiffness in the muscles of the shoulder girdle and upper arms and sometimes in the buttocks and thighs. The ESR is nearly always raised, sometimes to more than 100 mm in the first hour, and the alkaline phosphatase is occasionally raised. Treatment is with corticosteroids and the response may be very dramatic with the symptoms disappearing overnight. Some patients with temporal (cranial) arteritis,

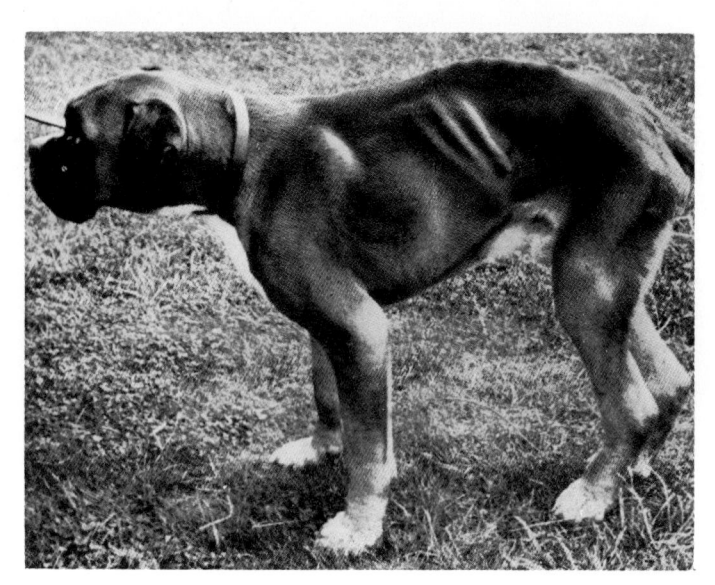

Fig. 14.6. Patient whose x-ray is shown in Fig. 5, before operation.

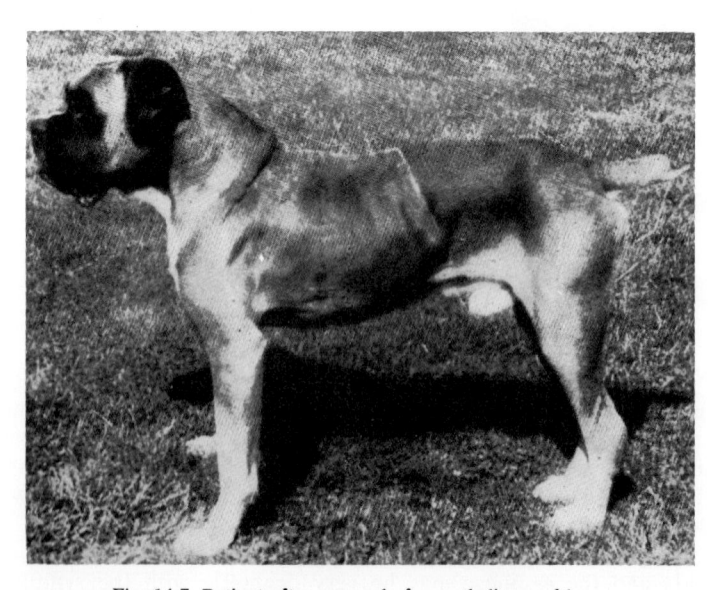

Fig. 14.7. Patient after removal of mesothelioma of lung.

an inflammatory condition of the cranial arteries, have symptoms similar to polymyalgia rheumatica before the arthritis develops, and this condition should always be considered in patients with the polymyalgia rheumatica syndrome. A definite diagnosis may be made by biopsy of a temporal artery. This shows characteristic histology with giant cells (so that the condition is sometimes called 'giant cell arteritis'). The biopsy also relieves the symptoms of headache. The importance of diagnosis is that the patient may go blind suddenly. Treatment with steroids prevents this.

15
Physiotherapy

Proper Use
Types of Physiotherapy
Exercises
  Basic forms
  Purpose
  Special types
    Postural
    Resisted
Hydrotherapy
Heat
Cold
Massage
Traction
Electrical Therapy
Dangers
Conclusion

Physiotherapy is the application of physical aids and forces to reduce pain and to maintain or improve function. It is a tremendously important factor in the management of the arthritic patient.

A recent analysis of the figures in the United Kingdom for the use of physiotherapy showed that 30% of the time was used to treat orthopaedic and rheumatological patients, 24% for trauma, 20% neurology, 13% chest diseases and 13% for other disabilities.

Proper Use

It is important that the skills of physiotherapists, who are in short supply, should be requested intelligently by doctors. A planned programme of treatment should be undertaken. This may be designed to overcome a specific disability. On the other hand it may be a programme of maintenance of function and morale, and the prevention of disability. A classic example of its value is in patients with ankylosing spondylitis.

Physiotherapy

The major aspect of treatment in these patients is by physiotherapy, and properly managed 85% of these patients never lose a day's work. It is the rheumatic disease above all others that must be treated with active exercise, and with the maintenance of mobility and posture.

Out-patient physiotherapy for rheumatic patients is of questionable value, particularly in the winter-time, when waiting for ambulances readily undoes any good that has been accomplished in the Physiotherapy Department. Some patients are keen to have physiotherapy as a social outing, but this is an abuse of scarce resources. Where sufferers are treated on an out-patient basis, they should be reviewed by the prescribing physician or surgeon after four weeks treatment, and earlier if they have responded satisfactorily, or if the physiotherapist requests an earlier review because the patient has deteriorated or developed other complications.

The amount of time spent in the Physiotherapy Department is always small compared with the working life of a patient, so that careful instructions for the continuance of aspects of therapy at home are vital. In the case of ankylosing spondylitis, for instance, it is not usually necessary for the patient to attend for regular treatment. It is our policy, however, that all such patients should receive careful instruction on one or two occasions from the physiotherapist about the regime of exercises that they should pursue at home. Advice may also be given about the most suitable beds and chairs they should use.

Types of Physiotherapy

A summary of many forms of physical therapy are shown in Table 15.1. It is seen that these fall into passive and active forms. The emphasis is on active therapy these days, and passive forms are often used merely as a prelude to active treatment.

Exercises

Basic forms

There are three basic forms of exercise:

(1) Totally 'passive' movements which, of course, are not really exercise by the patient but are done by the physiotherapist assisted by the nurse with the patient totally relaxed, because he is usually incapable of performing the movements himself. These movements are in *no* way forced and they are totally different from other forced manipulations which are normally only done at the express wish of the doctor concerned. During the acute phase of rheumatoid arthritis gentle passive movements may be used.

Physical Agent	Application	Effect
1. Exercise	Passive Active assisted Full free active Postural Resisted Special (e.g. PNF Bobath, Rood)	Improve mobility Increase strength Improve co-ordination Improve posture Enhance endurance
2. Water	Undercurrent massage Hubbard tank Deep pool	Local heat & massage Relax spasm Exercise without gravity Exercise against buoyancy of water
3. Heat	Moist heat Wax/oil baths Radiant heat Short wave diathermy Ultrasound Diapulse	Relief of pain Muscle relaxation Increase circulation Effect on connective tissues
4. Cold	Ice Cooling spray	Raise pain threshold Counter-irritation
5. Massage	Friction Vichy bath Deep connective tissue	Muscle relaxation Reduce oedema Counter-irritation
6. Traction	Stretching Manipulation Wedging	Separate surfaces Break adhesions Improve joint range Stretch contracted tissues
7. Electricity	Ion transfer Stimuli	Introduce ions locally Contract muscles

Table 15.1 A summary of forms of physiotherapy.

(2) Active assisted exercises aided by the operator when the patient, due to muscle weakness, is capable of doing only a small amount of joint movement himself. Assistance may be given by the operator himself or by springs, pulleys, or even water which acts as an uplift to the patient's limb.

(3) Full free active exercise performed by the patient totally unaided.

Physiotherapy 147

Purpose exercises

These are undertaken:
(1) To improve the range of movement of the joint, as for example restoring the mobility in a patient with periarthritis of the shoulder, or to improve the chest expansion of a patient with ankylosing spondylitis.
(2) To strengthen muscles and enhance endurance. The strength of muscles can be developed by exercising them against gradually increasing resistance. Muscles can be exercised against the resistance of gravity and by using lead weights, springs, or the manual resistance of the physiotherapist. To increase endurance light weights or medium resistance with a high repetition of the exercise are used. To increase power or strength heavy weights or maximum resistance are applied for a low number of repetitions.
(3) To improve co-ordination and posture. The scheme of exercises is adapted to the patient's condition, age, and occupation e.g. elderly housewife, young coal miner. For the severely disabled these would range from rolling over in bed, getting in and out of bed, standing and walking, to going up and down stairs.

It may be necessary to teach patients how to walk evenly on the floor, how to turn around with the aid of a stick after they have been in bed for a period, to walk on different types of surfaces (smooth and uneven), and to negotiate stairs.

Specific activities may be undertaken such as training them in getting on a bus step. We have the back of a bus, kindly donated by the West Yorkshire Bus Company for this purpose. A bus step is surprisingly high, and if a patient lives in the country we remove the step up to it because of the absence of kerbs in rural districts. The particular bus we use has side rails at a different height and has been so designed that the conductor cannot possibly help the patient to mount the step. In Leeds the Sixth Form of the Central High School undertook 'Project B.O.B.' (Back of Bus), in which they constructed apparatus which simulated the back of a bus and incorporated the vibration of a standing vehicle.

Where the patient is using an appliance such as crutches, a walking tripod, a walking stick, or a Zimmer walking frame, training will be required to teach him to use these devices properly. These should be adjusted to the individual patient's height.

Special types of exercise

(a) *Postural.* These exercises are often employed to preserve or restore the proper alignment of the spine and to encourage the normal effortless balance of the head, neck and shoulders, which often deteriorates rapidly following long debilitating illness or confinement to bed. This especially occurs in growing children. Deteriorating posture gives rise to increasing shearing and rotational stresses on the various segments of the spine and greater effort and resultant muscle fatigue must inevitably occur to prevent the body bending still further. Such exercises are important in back, neck and shoulder girdle pains which arise in the middle-aged patient in conditions such as cervical spondylosis or in younger patients with ankylosing spondylitis and rheumatoid arthritis.

(b) *Resisted.* Used primarily to strengthen muscles and increase joint range. These should be objectively graded and recorded, and the patient's capability reassessed regularly so that more resistance is added and maximal effort is called for from the patient.

It is important to emphasise that with all programmes of exercises, maintenance of these at home for definite periods each day is essential.

There are other specialised forms of physiotherapy, such as PNF (proprioceptive neuromuscular facilitation), Bobath and Rood techniques, and other mobilising and manipulative techniques. These are only occasionally used for rheumatic patients and their complexity is beyond the scope of this chapter.

Group exercises are most useful for rheumatic patients especially in the early wheel chair stage. They can prove enjoyable and stimulating.

Hydrotherapy

Some forms of hydrotherapy are sophisticated means of heat and massage. Vichy baths are one example and undercurrent baths are another. Invaluable help can be gained from treatment in the deep pool (or a Hubbard tank for those patients who may require treatment separately). The tank may be used when patients have a skin condition that may be distressing to other sufferers, or where their bowel or urinary problems necessitate a change of water after the treatment. A Hubbard tank may also be used if individualised therapy is particularly required. Many departments, however, would feel the tank is outmoded. The advantage of hydrotherapy is that the warmth of the water provides muscle relaxation, and the buoyancy of the water allows patients to do many things which it would not be possible for them to do outside the pool. Floats are used to support the patient in the water and to resist or assist movements. The treatment is particularly valuable for hip problems, and younger patients with osteoarthrosis may be able to postpone surgery on the hip following a course of hydrotherapy in the deep pool lasting as long as six weeks. The therapy

Physiotherapy

may also be useful for knee problems as part of rehabilitation following surgery on the knee, in the treatment of back problems, and the mobilisation of shoulders with restricted movement.

Some workers have advocated the drinking of waters! Spa therapy relies heavily on various types of hydrotherapy. The intensive treatment and careful programming of therapy that patients receive in such an environment is extremely beneficial. It is doubtless this approach rather than the magical properties of the waters (be they sulphur, radioactive, or whatever), that contributes to the progress of the patients.

Heat

This is given to relieve pain and relax muscles. It also increases the local circulation. Wax baths or oil baths are commonly used for treatment of rheumatoid hands and, less commonly, feet. We have designed a unit to be used for either purpose (Fig. 15.1). With wax

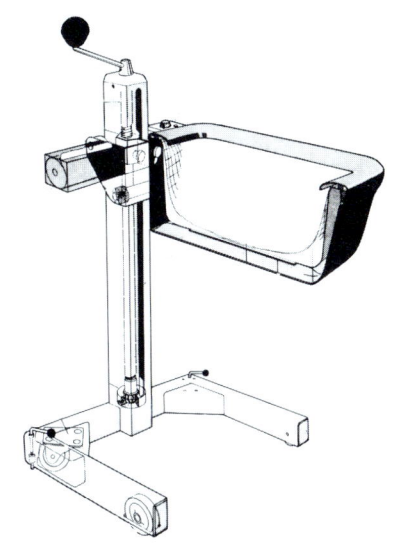

Fig. 15.1 An oil/wax bath for the treatment of hands or feet.

baths, the patient's hands are coated by dipping them in and out of the wax a number of times, allowing a layer of low melting point wax to solidify on the hands. They are then wrapped in grease-proof paper and a towel. The patient sits meditatively for 20 minutes. This should be followed by suitable hand and wrist exercises. Wax baths may be used at home, but it is important to warn the patient that the wax should not be heated directly in a pan, but rather in a stone jar container of water. In this way wax does not spill over on to the cooker with the possibility of fire. Radiant heat may be used for superficial heating, as in the cervico-brachial region when there are pains around the shoulder girdle. Heat may be given in the form of moisture, such as hot packs. We sometimes use mudpacks at our Department at Harrogate, in which mud is heated and put between cloths and then applied to areas such as a knee. It has the advantage that it can be moulded around the joint, that the heat is retained for a considerable period, and the weight of the mud may also help to overcome flexion deformities whilst the warmth is relaxing muscle spasm around the painful joint.

Deeper heat required for the treatment of osteoarthrosis of the hip or knee, is provided by short wave diathermy. Ultrasonic therapy and diapulse therapy are used for their effect on connective tissues, but further research is necessary before the value of these treatments can be assessed in relation to rheumatic diseases.

Cold

Crushed ice to make ice packs may be helpful for painful areas. It is said to work because it increases local circulation of the capsule, and may 'shunt' the blood into deeper structures, it reduces pain sensitivity, it relaxes muscle spasm, it diminishes muscle fatigue and therefore improves muscle strength. Sometimes a joint which has not responded to heat may improve with cold therapy. Ice is particularly valuable if swelling is present. Cooling sprays (containing 85% trichloromonofluoromethane and 15% dichlorodifluoromethane) are sometimes used, particularly for painful areas on the trunk, and they may be effective in post-herpetic neuralgia. It may well be that the spray works by counter-irritation. At home, the use of a 2lb bag of frozen peas, for the shoulder, or a 5lb bag for the knees is a useful re-useable method of applying cold.

Massage

Doubtless massage does aid muscle relaxation in certain situations, and may be particularly useful in pain around the shoulder girdle. It should be remembered, however, that it is time-consuming, and applied by a pleasant physiotherapist may become 'a drug of addiction'. Vichy baths are a sophisticated form of massage, in which the muscles are massaged whilst sprays of warm water are directed on to the affected part. If a physician feels that massage is indicated, he does well to give consideration to this being applied by a relative at home. Although it will obviously not be given with the skill of a trained therapist, it may benefit the patient. The benefit gained from many of the embrocations recommended are probably due partly to their counter-irritant effect and partly to the accompanying massage (regardless of the nature of the preparation). Deep connective tissue massage is a tiring, time-consuming mode of therapy, but it does seem to be of benefit in intractable cases of muscular pain, and has been claimed to have good results in systemic sclerosis and circulatory conditions such as Raynaud's disease.

Traction

Neck traction is commonly prescribed, although a controlled trial has not shown it to affect the natural course of neck pains. Low back pain which does not respond to a period of bed rest on a firm mattress with underlying boards, may be treated with pelvic traction or leg traction. Often this may work just by the enforced immobilisation, since the weights supplied are insufficient to distract bony structures in the spine. Manipulation may be used cautiously where a flexion contracture is not responding to simple measures, or in some cases of low back pain. Often this is done under anaesthesia by a clinician.

Wedge plastering to overcome a flexion deformity of the knee is in fact a form of stretching. The leg is encased in a plaster cylinder and a cut made in the plaster transversely across the popliteal fossa. The plaster is wedged open with a cork and the procedure repeated every few days. Caution must be taken not to produce a common peroneal (lateral popliteal) nerve palsy, or to produce pressure on the skin over the patella.

Electrical Therapy

The stimulus of muscles by faradism, where little active contraction can be obtained from a wasted muscle, is still sometimes used, and faradic foot baths are particularly useful in the stiff painful foot. Such stimulation should be used mainly in the early stage of muscle re-education to help initiate muscle action which the patient cannot perform himself. It should be discontinued when the patient can understand and initiate the movement himself. Exceptional cases occur where the patient is quite incapable of moving a joint himself, e.g. in hemiplegia or paraplegia where joint stiffness must be overcome and circulation maintained.

Ion transfer is a form of therapy largely discarded today. Renotin ionisations used to be performed for locally painful conditions. Forms of heat, such as short wave diathermy, are sometimes classified under this heading, as well as ultrasonic and diapulse therapy.

Dangers

Like all useful treatments, physiotherapy has its dangers. Burns may result from the application of heat. For this reason the sensitivity of the patient to warmth should be tested prior to the application of heat, or the patient should be watched with particular care, and the length of time of treatments not exceeded. It is essential that short wave diathermy should not be used when metallic implants have been inserted, otherwise the tissue around the implants will fry. Patients with epilepsy should not have short wave diathermy.

Exercise in active arthritis may provoke an exacerbation and must be used gently and cautiously. Likewise, enthusiastic but ill-advised efforts at premature manipulation of joints with restricted movement may cause an exacerbation of symptoms and aggravate the situation. Exercises have often been advocated for protruded intervertebral discs, but recent work in Scandinavia, in which the pressure in discs has been measured during various physiotherapy manoeuvres, demonstrates that these may also cause a worsening of the situation (Fig. 15.2).

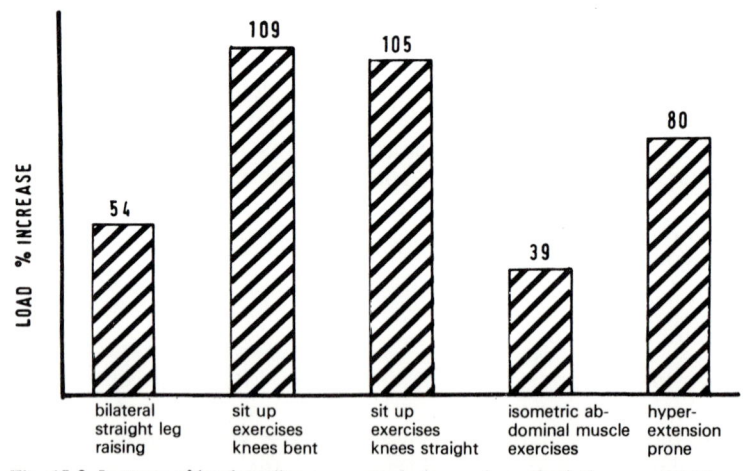

Fig. 15.2. Increase of lumbar disc pressures during various physiotherapy activities.

Conclusion

Physiotherapy is plainly a most valuable adjunct to treatment of patients with rheumatism and arthritis. It is not without its dangers, however, and must be used intelligently and carefully. It is emphasised that a planned programme is required, that treatment should not go on ad infinitum, and that one of the most important aspects is the training given for the continuation of therapy at home. Passive therapy aimed at relaxing muscle spasm and relieving pain has a role to play, but the most important aspects are active treatments.

16
Occupational Therapy

Remedial Programme
  Joint protection
Specific Programme
  Fingers
  Wrists
  Elbows
  Shoulders
  Ankles
  Knees
  Hips
Assessment of Patients
  Occupation
Severe Disability
An Illustrative Disease
Splintage
Nursing
  Bed heights
  Bathing
  Easy chairs
  Wheelchairs

For too long occupational therapy has been considered in terms of patients making cuddly toys to while away the time. The skills of the occupational therapist are vital in the rehabilitation of arthritic sufferers. The occupational therapist is concerned in this total rehabilitation with assessment in the activities of daily living with a view to helping their situation by means of re-training the patient, strengthening the functions which remain, making suitable modifications to implements that they use, and in their settlement at home and at work. The occupational therapist is also concerned to devise a remedial programme for the patient. At times this may include diversional therapy, but it is a very small part of the overall work.

Many nurses are excellent in their job of nursing but insufficiently educated in rehabilitation. So much more can be achieved whilst an in-patient, if the nursing staff are operating at the same level of activity with the patient as that being aimed at by the physiotherapist and occupational therapist. Information about this must be passed on to the ward staff to prevent the patient becoming totally dependent on the nursing staff and only active in the physiotherapy and occupational therapy departments. The patient is otherwise deprived of practice, mobilisation and exercise tolerance.

Remedial Programme

The overall philosophy governing the remedial programme devised by the occupational therapists is that of purposeful activity (Fig. 16.1). This must be done in consultation with the medical, nursing and

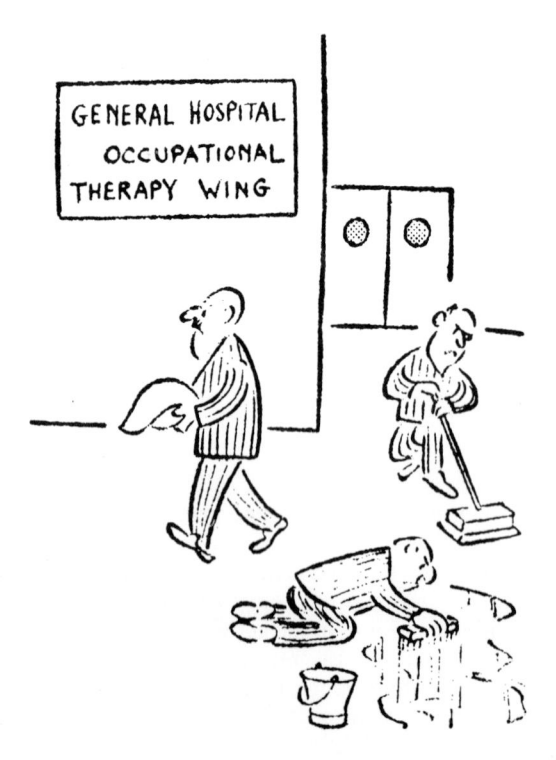

Fig. 16.1. Purposeful activity from an occupational therapy department.

physiotherapy staff members. Indeed, the programme should be set up as a joint venture with the physiotherapist and ward staff. Ideally the occupational therapy and physiotherapy departments in hospital should be adjacent, so that there is social as well as functional liaison. We often find in our Unit that the occupational therapist is able to discuss a particular problem where the skills of the physiotherapist will help to remedy the situation, and vice versa. The patients' activities should be co-ordinated with the nursing staff to ensure those activities which the patient should be doing are done by the patients; that help is given where required and not when the patients should be doing it themselves. In this way the patient can work towards maximum independence and increase their tolerance to exercise. Consultation with the patient is always rewarding. The patient has often found a way of doing an activity which can be passed on to another. Patients tend to learn better from fellow sufferers than from staff. In considering the programme the type of arthritis must be recognised and the activity of the disease determined. Patients with ankylosing spondylitis require a vigorous course of therapy, whilst rheumatoid arthritis in the subacute phase requires cautious activity lest there should be a flare up of symptoms. The maximum range of movement of joints consistent with the disease must be encouraged.

Joint protection

Deforming positions and stresses should be avoided. For instance, pinching exercises may exert an undue force at the metacarpophalangeal joints of patients with rheumatoid arthritis, producing dislocation of the joints. In a pinch grip the ulnar deviating force exerted at the metacarpophalangeal joints is ten times that exerted at the finger tips. For this reason it is better to use therapy involving the handling of larger circular objects, rather than small ones. Alternatively, the metacarpophalangeal joints may be kept in a good position by an appropriate splint.

The joints should be used in the most favourable direction and the strongest joints available should be utilised for the activity employed. Activities should be avoided that maintain one position for long periods. No activity should be attempted that cannot be stopped immediately, and pain should be respected. It is often nature's warning signal to desist. The length and frequency of periods of therapy must be adjusted with the patient's disease and stage of activity. Likewise associated disabilities, such as heart disease, have to be taken into account. The emotional needs of the patient must not be neglected. In devising a programme the patient's talents and previous skills must not be ignored and the development of latent talent encouraged.

In protecting damaged joints the use of the body must be carefully considered. This may involve sitting to work and using both hands. Other parts of the body may also be used. For example, a lever may be operated with the forearm rather than deformed painful fingers. Needless motion should be eliminated, and thought must be given to how gravity and momentum can be made to work for the patient, so that objects can sometimes be slid rather than moved. Alternatively the effects of gravity are avoided by the use of appropriate slings. Prolonged holding is not usually desirable.

Specific Programme

Various crafts may be used for specific joint mobilisation.

Fingers

To encourage flexion, paper cutting, puppetry, basketry, weaving, needlework, knotting, leather lacing, may all be employed. To encourage extension, block printing, certain types of pottery, knotting, finger painting and braid weaving may be used. Other activities may include typing, sanding blocks, making coathangers and pin and wire pictures, stool seating and adapted games (e.g. bobbin draughts).

Wrists

Extension may be encouraged by use of the printing press, book binding, lathe work, weaving, block printing, wood carving, linoleum block cutting and sanding. Flexion is required in book binding, carving, braid weaving and basketry. The wire twisting machine encourages flexion and extension of the wrists.

Elbows

Flexion is used in woodworking, leather working, basketry, knotting, weaving, winding yarn and stool seating. Extension may be encouraged with printing, planing, woodwork, coping saw projects, braid weaving and hammering (although in the last the jarring on the joints must be considered in relation to the activity). Pronation is used in screw driving and crocheting. Likewise supination is employed in stool seating.

Shoulders

Elevation may be accomplished by weaving, rug loom work, basketry with pual spokes and knotting. Flexion is encouraged by printing,

Occupational Therapy

woodworking and knotting; abduction by leather lacing, basketry, weaving and knotting; rotation by winding wool and wheel weaving.

Ankles

Flexion and extension are the main movements required here and these may be accomplished by the use of foot powered lathes, foot powered fretsaw cutter, potter's wheel, and sewing machine.

Knees

Flexion is used in fretsaw cutting with a foot operated machine, and a floor loom. An electrically controlled bicycle saw may also be used for knees and hips. Likewise extension may be accomplished by two activities, and by the potter's wheel.

Hips

The same types of machinery used for the ankles and knees accomplishes many of the movements required at the hip. Sometimes one finds a patient with skill on the organ and this is useful for abduction of the hips.

Assessment of Patients

In our Units all patients with rheumatic diseases who are admitted to hospital have an assessment in the activities of daily living by the occupational therapist which is included in the case record. The assessment is in three main areas. First the personal activities, such as toilet, feeding, bathing, washing and dressing. Secondly, domestic activities such as cooking, washing up, sewing and laundry. Thirdly, problems involved in travelling to work, and carrying it out. Where there are problems in personal and domestic activities, retraining may be necessary.

In addition, modification of the home may be required by altering the levels of tables, cookers, beds and chairs. Rails may be required to help a patient rise from the lavatory or the bath, or to negotiate stairs. One occupational therapy student in her final examination wrote: 'Every rheumatoid patient is helped by a bar in the toilet!' It may be necessary to provide a raised toilet seat, and this is one of the most welcome provisions (Fig. 16.2). Likewise a bath seat may help the patient and a non-slip bath mat is often necessary. The provision of a shower may overcome bathing problems, although in a survey in Leeds showers were not popular as an alternative to baths, possibly because of the beneficial effect of being immersed in hot water.

It may be impossible for patients to dress or to do their hair (Fig. 16.3). For these and other difficulties aids can be provided. These should be characterised by simplicity, usefulness and speed of provision. Essential for their success is a good assessment of the patient and knowledge of how to cope with the problem, a good rapport between the patient and the team managing the patient, a good assessment of

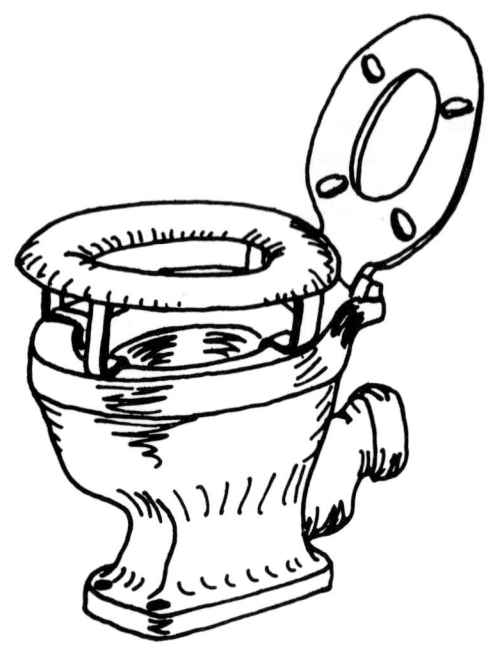

Fig. 16.2. Raised toilet seat.

the total situation and training and persistence where overcoming the problem is a new experience for the patient. Many useful aids are made by patients themselves in the occupational therapy department or the remedial workshop. Typical of useful aids are long handled combs (Fig. 16.4) rubazote handles to cutlery to enable the patient to grasp them (Fig. 16.5) a long handled shoe horn, a long handle to a sponge for back-washing, and tap turners. Holes cut in the kitchen table to hold mixing bowls or non-slip plastic mesh may be valuable. A pick-up stick (Fig. 16.6) to enable patients with restricted movement at the hips or knees enables objects to be retrieved from the floor. It is also useful as an aid to dressing.

The height of chairs may be important. The patient with rheumatoid arthritis flops down into a chair and has difficulty in getting up from a

Occupational Therapy

low chair. For that reason in our out-patient department and wards we have specially high chairs with a seat height of 19½ inches, and wooden side arms to help the patients lever themselves out. If the chair is too low to enable patients to rise without help, they are totally dependent. The right height of chair may make the difference between dependency and independence.

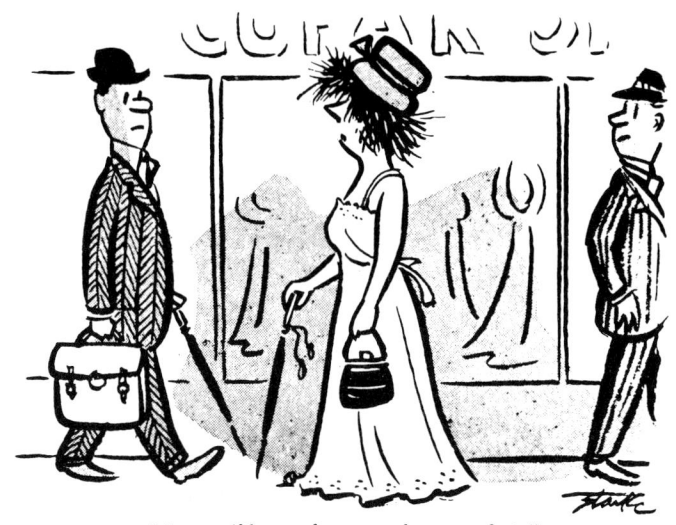

"*Impossible to dress or do your hair*"

Fig. 16.3. Some problems for arthritic patients.

Where one hand is particularly disabled, a series of aids to help the patient cope may be required. For instance, a mounted potato peeler, or a potato board with spikes that fix the potato while it is being peeled with the relatively good hand. A combined knife/fork may also make eating much easier, although this is more often used by hemiplegic patients.

Patients should be instructed in ways to hold things that will be the least damaging to their joints. For instance, plates should not be held at the edge but with the hand underneath providing a wider, firmer base. Similarly, heavy pans should be held underneath with one hand where possible, and the other hand palm upwards holding the handle. Alternatively light pans may be advocated. Heavy books should not be held dragging rheumatoid fingers into ulnar deviation, but put on a book rest.

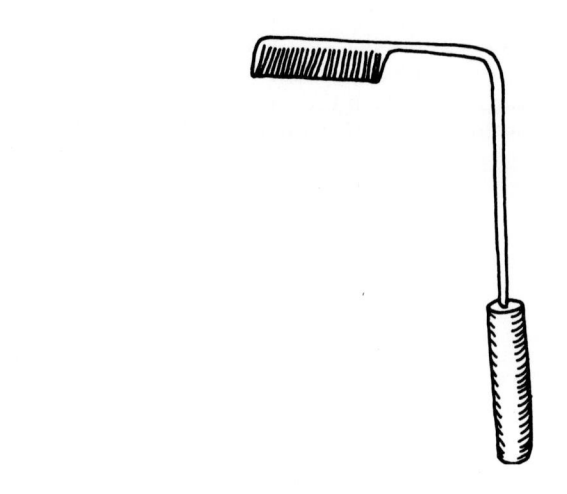

Fig. 16.4. Long handled combs.

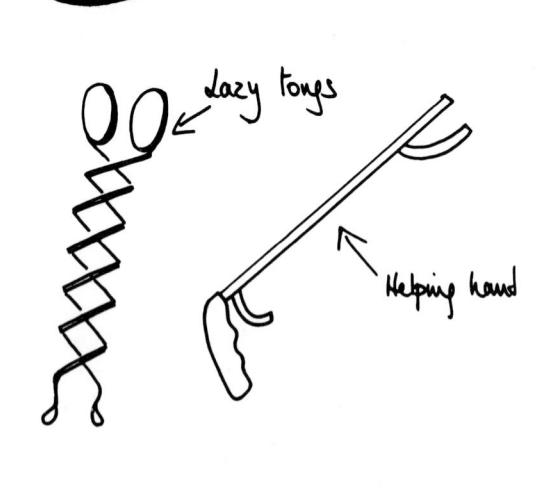

Fig. 16.5. Enlarged handles of cutlery.

Fig. 16.6. Pick-up sticks.

Occupation

As far as working is concerned, the principles are that forces required should be reduced as much as possible. This may mean changing the method of doing a job. Sometimes our occupational therapist visits a factory with a bioengineer or remedial workshop technician to suggest to the management minor modifications that will help the patient—and often incidentally speed up production! At times harmful activities can be eliminated, or on other occasions specialised equipment may help the patient to cope with the situation.

As far as the work place is concerned, sometimes a special work centre is required for the disabled patient. Work height should be comfortable and the total work area in easy reach. Likewise the tools and supplies should be easily seen and reached. The equipment and supplies should be positioned for an easy flow of work. In terms of tools and equipment, ideally multi-purpose tools should be used. The handles should be easy to grasp and controls should be easy to reach and operate. It is best to try and get the patient back to the firm in which they have been working for some time, since the management will be the most sympathetic to the patient's problems and appreciate his potentialities. Where re-training is required, assessment at an Industrial Rehabilitation Unit may be arranged in the first instance, through the Disablement Resettlement Officer, with whom the therapist should have a good liaison.

Severe Disability

With the severely disabled patient, sticks and crutches may be necessary (Fig. 16.7).

Assessment of mobility is of great importance. Many patients will require no aids. Others may require a walking stick which should be cut to a comfortable height. Fisher sticks have a moulded handle which fits neatly into the palm. Tripods and quadrapods are more often used by hemiplegics. Axillary crutches are a useful aid for the short periods of use required in orthopaedics, but are generally unsuitable for long term use. Gutter crutches, in which the forearm is placed in the gutter distributing the weight over a wide area, are of more use particularly to arthritic patients with poor grip. Severely disabled patients, especially those with predominant involvement of their hips and knees, may require walking frames. One version is now available which allows walking up and down stairs.

Most rheumatologists go to great lengths to keep patients out of wheelchairs. If these prove necessary, careful assessment is needed if the correct type is to be prescribed. The need for such extras as ball bearing arm supports should also be assessed. Unfortunately several of the more sophisticated chairs are not available through the NHS and must be privately purchased. It is especially important that these are purchased after skilled assessment rather than skilled advertising. Ramps in and out of the home may also aid mobility.

Aid with transport is usually restricted to those who require a car to get to and from work. This may take the form of financial assistance towards the licence or modification of the patient's own car. Assessment for motorised transport is undertaken by specialists working at Artificial Limb and Appliance Centres.

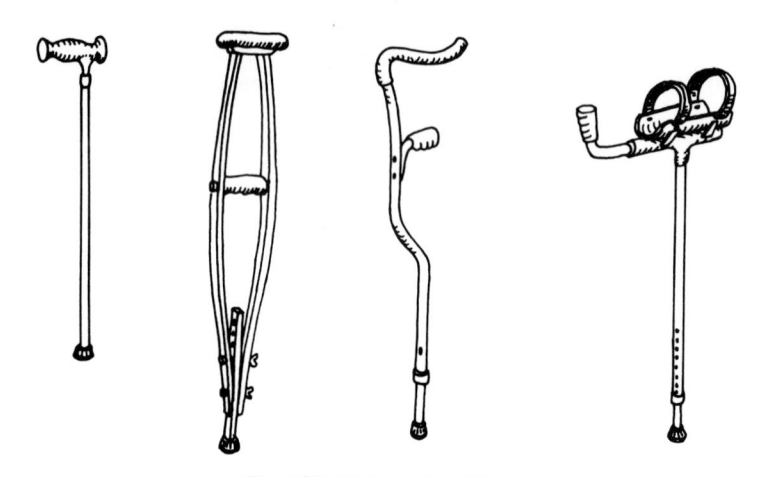

Fig. 16.7. Sticks and crutches.

An Illustrative Disease

The role of occupational therapy in the management of ankylosing spondylitis is a good example of the value of this discipline. With these patients, in all activities a good posture must be encouraged to prevent flexion deformities of the upper part of the spine, and in employment care must be taken to ensure the seat is at the correct height and distance from the work. It is, however, important to remember that some flexion of the spine is necessary, and a spine which is too straight can be a worse handicap than a flexion deformity. Weaving on an upright loom is a useful activity, encouraging good posture. The 'stand-sit' chair is useful, since it is high, and the adjustable bicycle type of seat does not prevent hip movement (Fig. 16.8). Hip movements are obtained at the loom by depression of the two foot pedals using flexion and extension of each hip alternately. These pedals may be adjusted sideways to produce abduction and adduction of the hips.

Other treadle machines may be used at this stage of treatment, e.g. lathes, fret-saws and sawing machines will help to keep the hips moving if the patient uses them in a standing position or with a high chair, but care must be taken with posture since the work involved often encourages stooping.

In the rare advanced case a programme of interesting light activities may provide stimulation and avoid depression. Activities in a standing

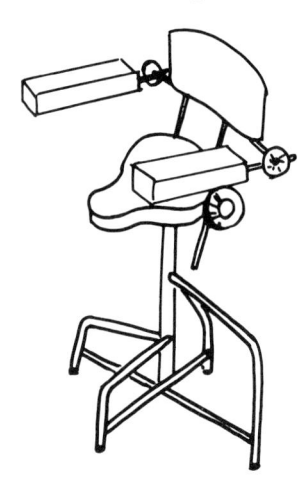

Fig. 16.8. 'Stand-sit' chair, showing the bicycle type seat; note adjustable height of seat and position of arms.

position are best, since sitting is uncomfortable, and in this way muscle power of the legs is improved. Painting and drawing may be valuable for some patients, care being given to the height and angle of the easel. If the patient is liable to lose his balance in this position, he may be placed in a sling fastened to a stable piece of furniture. Since the patient may have restricted head movement, work and tools must be carefully placed and the type of painting wisely chosen, since large drawings or wide areas of painting will be difficult to manage. The desk should be wide enough to allow the work to be moved rather than the head.

With advanced disease it is particularly important to ascertain the home conditions and assess the patient in terms of daily living. The main problem of the spondylitic patient is often reaching the floor. For some, if the hips are stiff but not totally immobile, there may be a way of bending down with one leg outstretched, or by bending backwards with the knees bent, while holding on to the furniture. If knee and ankle movements are good then kneeling should be used regularly.

Should this not be possible, there are several types of long-handled tongs and reaching aids which are available or can be made.

Another problem is that of reaching the feet for putting on shoes, socks, pants and trousers, and washing the feet. Many patients find that by lying on their beds on one side and by bending the opposite knee they can reach their feet sufficiently well to perform these tasks. Alternatively they may lie on their back with their legs in the air. If the knees are stiff, particular problems are encountered. Some patients manage with the aid of tongs and reaching aids. If these fail then aids to assist putting on socks may be issued such as sock/stocking aids and elastic shoe laces, long-handled shoe horns or a shoe board. A long-handled sponge may serve for washing the feet. Two long tapes with suspender fasteners on the ends can be used for a simple type of sock aid and for pulling on pants and trousers. Removing a garment (particularly a heavy jacket or overcoat) can be as difficult as putting it on and dressing sticks may be valuable. The sticks are made from a piece of dowelling of appropriate length, one end of which has a long finger stall over it and the other has a hook to help with pulling on clothes. An ordinary walking stick may serve the same purpose. It may be helpful to hang a coat in a suitable position over the back of an upright chair to allow the arms to slip in the sleeves easily. Bathing may prove a severe problem and the installation of a shower may be necessary. Other bath aids may be useful—these include a bath seat, a non-slip bath mat and a slider. A raised toilet seat may be necessary with a handrail firmly fixed to the wall. The height of other seats require adjustments. For patients with widespread ankylosis we have developed an armchair with a motor-driven mechanism to tilt the seat to overcome the problem of getting in and out of the chair.

A female spondylitic requires retraining in the kitchen. Long-handled implements enable her to reach the floor. A trolley may be used as a walking aid. If the wheels run too freely a type of automatic brake may be fixed which causes the brakes to come into action when a patient relaxes. Equipment, cupboards, sink and refrigerator require adjusting to the appropriate height. Where ankylosis is widespread patients may have difficulty in managing their job, especially if it is arduous, so that retraining in another occupation may be necessary. A course in an Industrial Rehabilitation Unit may be beneficial for this purpose.

Braces are seldom indicated, except in advanced cases. Of themselves they will not correct posture and are to be deprecated in the early phase.

Where symptoms are produced by residual movement at the junction of two stiff segments immobilisation rather than exercise may be required but this is unusual. The same may be true in certain types of atypical spondylitis.

Splintage

The question of splintage is discussed in Chapter 17. The provision of such splints often falls to the lot of the occupational therapist, particularly with the newer materials that can be moulded in a hospital environment, and do not require high temperatures to work them. Splints may be used to rest inflamed joints, to overcome deformities, to allow function by maintaining a joint in a satisfactory position. Some examples of these are shown in Figs. 17.1-17.5.

The patient needs to be encouraged to wear splints and the occupational therapist often has the responsibility of seeing the patient knows how to put them on and take them off, and when they should be worn.

Nursing

In many hospitals there is an inadequate establishment of occupational therapy posts and some of the procedures discussed above may be undertaken by the physiotherapist or by the nursing staff. Even with a full establishment however, an integrated programme must be undertaken both in hospital and in the community. The following are a few additional details which help nurses in the vital role they have to play as members of the therapeutic (rehabilitation) team.

Bed heights

Many hospital beds are now adjustable but frequently they are not used for the patients' benefit.

Bathing

Nurses and district nurses tend to do what is safe or quick. Wards do not always have bathing aids the patient could be learning to use. Instead patients are often helped by two nurses. District nurses from pressure of time prefer to bed-bath, whereas immersing in hot water may be beneficial.

Easy chairs

Patients should sometimes have the chair suited to their degree of mobility. There is a tendency for some nurses to be happier if the patient cannot get up and walk because this ensures safety. The patient then has to rely on help when requiring to walk about.

Wheelchairs

It is questionable whether the assessment of type required and training in their use should be the sole prerogative of the occupational therapist. It ought to be very much part of the rehabilitation programme, yet nurses do not have specialised knowledge of wheelchairs.

17

Rehabilitation

Scope of Rehabilitation
Factors affecting Rehabilitation
The Patient
  Occupational therapy
  Health visiting
  Physical therapy
  Splintage
  Shoes
  Chiropody
Education of the Patient
The Environment

Scope of Rehabilitation

A national survey of handicapped and impaired in Great Britain showed that one in 13 persons over the age of 16 is not only impaired (i.e. has some disability) but is also handicapped by his impairment.

In a local survey of Leeds the figures were similar. One in nine persons over the age of 16 had mental, physical or sensory impairment and of these 2% suffered from rheumatoid arthritis and 26% had some other form of arthritis or rheumatism. 58% of the handicapped and impaired were over the age of 65 years, and one in five had difficulty with mobility.

In terms of the national economy the rheumatic diseases are of great importance, accounting for 37 million days lost annually from work. This represents several times the amount lost from all industrial stoppages. Moreover, from an individual's point of view, affliction by arthritis may well mean that he slides down the economic scale. The problem may be acute as with an intervertebral disc protrusion or it may be prolonged as in rheumatoid arthritis or osteoarthrosis.

Factors affecting Rehabilitation

Not only is there a great difference between various rheumatic diseases, but a single disease may exhibit a wide spectrum of manifestations. Thus, rheumatoid arthritis may be a shortlived episode with no recurrence or it may pursue an inexorable downhill course leading over a period of years to crippling. Frequently deterioration is erratic and unpredictable so that repeated modifications of life-style are required. On the other hand, with ankylosing spondylitis a generally optimistic prognosis can be given. Again, osteoarthrosis may involve only one joint and pose an isolated problem in an otherwise healthy patient, a problem which may be solved, for instance, by local surgery such as a total hip replacement. Not only the number of joints affected but their distribution modifies rehabilitation. An involved wrist which is maintained in a functional position is little disability, but pain and limited movement in weightbearing joints limit the activities of the patient. In certain occupations (e.g. in carpentry) involvement of the elbow may pose considerable problems, and the involvement of both shoulder and elbow may make it impossible for patients to reach the back of their hair or do up garments at the back, and may prevent jobs involving lifting. Where complications of the primary illness occur, such as the involvement of organs other than joints, discussed in an earlier chapter rehabilitation may become much more difficult.

Adequate treatment in the early stages is of vital importance in a disease like ankylosing spondylitis to prevent flexion deformities developing. It has not been proven that adequate early treatment affects the course of rheumatoid arthritis, but there can be little doubt that it is important for early acute cases to be hospitalised, not only to promote a remission of the active disease, but also for the patient to become acclimatised to the discipline of rest plasters and exercises designed to prevent deformity.

The importance of occupational factors is illustrated by the fact that those with sedentary jobs lose far less time from work due to arthritic disorders than those engaged in manual tasks.

Age is an important factor. With advancing years the number of patients with arthritic conditions on the Handicapped Register increases dramatically. Older patients also have more difficulty in learning new skills.

There are particular problems in the young. The young housewife who is unable to pick up or deal with her young children is at a serious disadvantage and the physical demands of the young family are heavy. This must be taken into account in family planning, even when there is no evidence that pregnancy actually modifies the disease process. If one suspects that a patient may not be able to cope with his present job in ten years' time, retraining should be considered, for at this stage retraining and re-employment are accomplished relatively easily. Once the patient has reached the age of 50 the employment market is such that, however well retrained the disabled person is, he is unlikely to find alternative employment.

The personality of the arthritic patient may be of importance in rehabilitation. There is no evidence of any unusual personality before the disease begins in most of these conditions, although there has been a suggestion of a 'periarthritic personality' in those suffering from periarthritis of the shoulder. A recent study in our department has shown that more of these patients suffer from insomnia before the disease develops than in a control group. Understandably in patients with rheumatoid arthritis anxiety commonly develops over the course of the disease and depression is frequent. Interestingly, it is the patients with mild to moderate disease who have the greatest anxiety and therefore careful attention must be paid to this aspect.

The support of family and friends is of great importance to the arthritic patient, especially when mobility is threatened. In a recent study of the impact on family life of young married women with rheumatoid arthritis, we have found the majority (80%) of these women drive themselves needlessly hard and require careful explanation of the life-style they should adopt. The greatest stress in not understanding the disease occurred in those patients who developed rheumatoid arthritis after marriage, particularly during the first two years of marriage. A feeling of guilt and the fear of being a burden interestingly occurred mostly in those with the best function, with the fewest eroded joints, with no children and in the earliest years of marriage.

The Patient

The use of drugs and surgery in the treatment of rheumatic disorders is dealt with elsewhere in this book. It is important that the disease should be seen in functional terms, however. For instance, morning stiffness may be the only problem preventing the patient returning to work and could be ameliorated by appropriate drugs.

Certain specific problems developing during the course of the disease may require the help of a specialist unit (e.g. flexion deformities of the knees, or in severe cases where there is a danger of the patient becoming immobilised). Gains may sometimes appear to be small, but they may make the difference between independence and dependence. Some of the problems affecting mobility may be involvement of the hips, often with flexion deformity and painful limitation of movement in all directions, flexion deformities of the knees, disease of the ankles and metatarso-phalangeal subluxation. Flexion deformities of the knees can usually be overcome by serial plastering, but involvement to this degree of hips is rarely relieved except by surgery. Overcoming flexion deformity of the hip by teaching the patient prone lying may prove helpful in postponing surgery. This is particularly important in the younger patient.

Occupational therapy

It may be of value to have a full assessment of those activities of daily living which the patient is finding difficult by an Occupational Therapist, either at home or in a hospital department, with a view to solving the problems raised. Their role is discussed in Chapter 16.

Health visiting

A Health Visitor may likewise be able to provide an overall assessment of the situation in the home. In a study we have undertaken, with two Health Visitors as a part of the team of an in-patient rehabilitation unit, the value of the Health Visitor was unquestionably shown. The bridge between the hospital and home and subsequent support of patients proved invaluable. Immediately on discharge she helped the patient at a time of insecurity and reinforced the instructions given in hospital. Further needs were ascertained as the patient came to terms with the home environment and the Health Visitor helped provide them.

Physical therapy

The aims of physical therapy are to relieve pain, to strengthen muscles and to improve the mobility of joints. For instance, all patients with ankylosing spondylitis should be taught a regime of exercises in the physiotherapy department which they should continue at home for many years; it may be necessary to check on these from time to time. It is important that these patients should maintain a good spinal posture throughout the day at work and in bed at night, and time should be spent in giving and reinforcing these instructions. In widespread disease the likely value of outpatient therapy must be balanced against the tiring effects of long waits for transport and bumpy ambulance journeys. If physiotherapy is indicated in these patients it is often best conducted on an in-patient basis, particularly where a deep pool is available. Hydrotherapy in the deep pool is particularly valuable for the treatment of weightbearing joints or when several joints are affected. Consideration should be given to whether the patient's desk, chair and bed help or hinder the preservation of good posture. These aspects are discussed in Chapter 14.

Splintage

The principles have been discussed in Chapter 16. Splints are readily made and are relatively cheap. Newer plastic materials have meant that cosmetically acceptable and lightweight splints are now available where long term use is required. It is important that the patient should have these renewed when necessary, and have fresh ones made if an alteration in the disease has made the wearing of a previous splint uncomfortable. When plaster splints are applied, the nurse should check the colour of the limb distal to the plaster, note the appearance of swelling and report any symptoms suggesting constriction of vessels with impairment of circulation. If the plaster is too tight it should be removed. It may also rub a small area and the plaster should be modified or removed immediately, since the skin of rheumatoid patients is easily damaged and heals slowly. It may suffice as a temporary measure to prevent rubbing by inserting sponge rubber or by wetting the edge of the plaster and altering its shape. Some examples of splints are shown in Figs. 17.1-17.4.

Flexion deformities of the knees may be overcome by serial plastering, in which the leg is encased in plaster with the knee in maximum extension for five to seven days. The plaster is then removed and a new plaster applied with the knee in further extension (Fig. 17.5). To overcome muscle spasm and allow greater extension of the knee intravenous diazepam may be given during the procedure. Wedge plastering may be used. This has been discussed in Chapter 15.

A third technique is that in which a cuffed plaster is put around the thigh and above the ankle. A rod projects from the upper plaster and is linked by a chain to a hook on the lower plaster. The chain is shortened from day to day. In a trial of three methods of straightening knees which we undertook, this proved the most effective. However, the procedure sometimes gave discomfort due to the difficulty of keeping the plaster cuff on the thigh in position and due to pressure on the patella of the metal rod. Cuffed plasters around a back slab are an alternative method of serial plastering. The advantage is that the knee is kept exposed, and injections of local hydrocortisone can be given if required during the period of straightening.

Shoes

For many patients the provision of shoes made-to-measure is a great boon. In a survey of patients who had been provided with such footwear in our clinic we found that all the men and 87% of the women were well satisfied with these. We avoid the use of the term 'surgical shoes' because it conjures up the image of big black boots whereas attractive

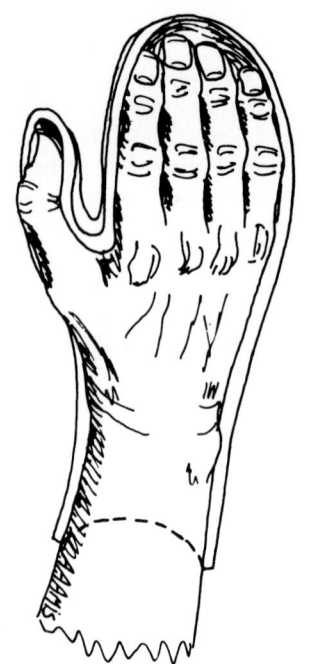

Fig. 17.1. Hand splint to rest the hand at night.

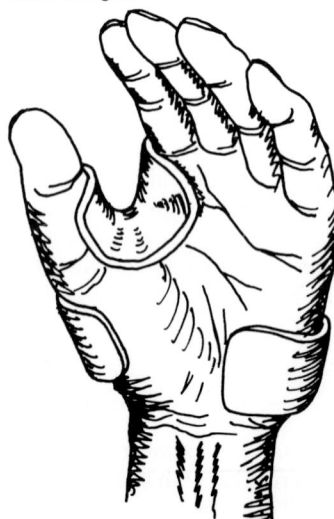

Fig. 17.2. Wrist splint.

Fig. 17.3. Opponens splint for thumb (view from palm).

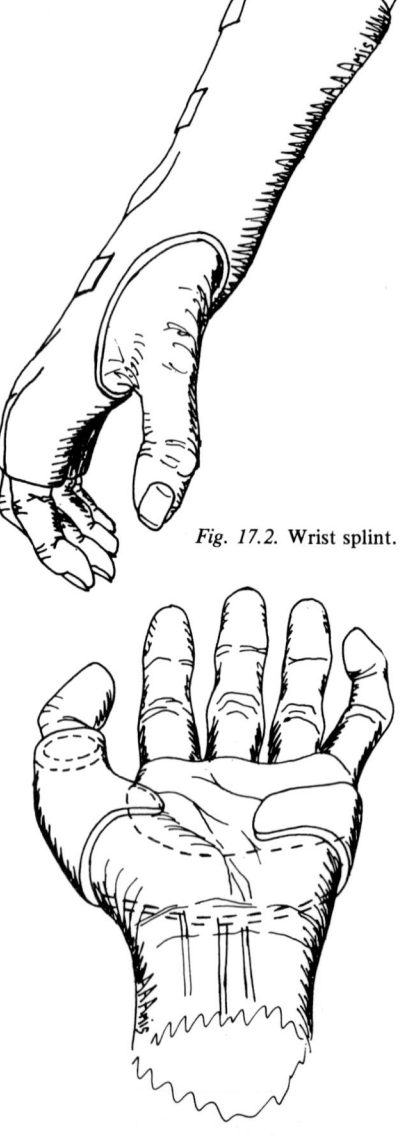

Fig. 17.4. Opponens splint for thumb (view to show how it fits on the dorsum of the hand).

shoes are now made. In the early stages of rheumatoid arthritis metatarsal insoles, metatarsal bars on the outside of the shoes, and boots instead of shoes for both men and women with ankle and subtalar pain may be adequate to provide relief. Later a below-knee caliper with double iron may be required for subtalar involvement in rheumatoid arthritis.

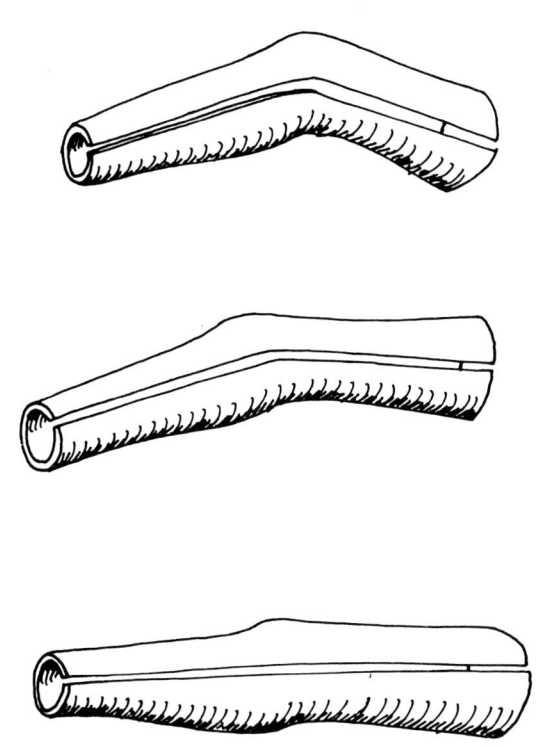

Fig. 17.5. Serial splints for a knee, used to overcome a flexion-deformity.

Chiropody

This is a frequently overlooked requirement for these patients. In a survey of rheumatic patients in our department half required chiropody. Women need it more than men.

Education of the Patient

In our survey of married women with rheumatoid arthritis the majority drove themselves too hard. Points that required particular explanation were the general effects of rheumatoid arthritis, how to adjust their level of activity and how to cope with life. Patients rarely retain much information imparted at a single interview. It may be helpful to repeat advice to the patient and extend it to the spouse also, particularly where longterm illness requires much family support.

To supplement the explanation to the patient the Arthritis and Rheumatism Council has produced a series of excellent booklets for patients, which are available to medical practitioners. These deal with rheumatoid arthritis, osteoarthrosis, ankylosing spondylitis, gout, and lumbar disc problems. There is also a series of booklets available for purchase by patients from the Arthritis and Rheumatism Council, Faraday House, 8-10 Charing Cross Road, London WC2H 0HN. These comprise 'Your Garden and your Rheumatism', 'Your Home and Your Rheumatism', and 'Marriage, Sex and Arthritis' (price 10p each). A number of useful books have also been published in the popular press dealing with rheumatic complaints. A recent one is that of Jayson and Dixon (1974) on 'Rheumatism and Arthritis; what they are and what you should know about them', published by Pan Books. The British Rheumatism and Arthritis Association provides patients with information, advice and practical aids.

The Environment

Difficulty in gripping and diminution of power are frequent disabilities in patients with rheumatoid arthritis and therefore certain aids may be required, such as: tap turners, door handles, tin openers, and modification of the handles of various implements. These are discussed in more detail in Chapter 16. Some modifications such as Mannoy tableware are specifically designed for the arthritic patient. It should be emphasised, however, that minor modifications of normal implements will often suffice to overcome disability. This may mean the widening or angulation of a handle (e.g. of comb) with rubazote. In patients with osteoarthrosis of the hip their lives can be greatly helped by chiropody, a pickup stick, a stocking aid or a walking stick. Certain patients with rheumatic disorders may require aids to mobility ranging from a walking stick to motorised transport. In rheumatoid disease where crutches are required the involvement of the arms may require the use of gutter rather than axillary crutches. Some patients also find that to angulate the end of the crutch may give added confidence. Often large handles are required. The clinical background of these problems is discussed in Chapters 3 and 6.

Where straps are required on appliances or on clothing, buckles should be avoided in patients with hand involvement, and velcro used instead. When wheelchairs are being ordered it is worth considering roller bearing arm supports where shoulders are weak. Otherwise aids to mobility follow the general pattern.

In returning the patient to work the help of the Disablement Resettlement Officer is invaluable and the patient may benefit from assessment at an Industrial Rehabilitation Unit, perhaps progressing to vocational training. The patient with ankylosing spondylitis rarely requires redirection in his employment, but certain jobs, such as that of a garage mechanic are unsuitable. The patient with rheumatoid arthritis has particular problems because of the exacerbations from which he may suffer over the years. For this reason strenuous efforts must be made to keep the patient's job where he has a sympathetic employer. Patients have to be assessed individually; there are times when a trained woman should be advised to undertake a sedentary job and employ domestic help rather than remain at home. The Community Services may be invaluable. The most greatly valued is that of a home help, and the provisions most frequently made by Local Authorities for patients at home are raised toilet seats, rails in the lavatory and bathroom, bath seats and non-slip bath mats. The Electricity Board and Gas Board will modify taps on cookers to permit the arthritic patient to manipulate these more easily. Telephones may also be modified. The Occupational Therapist may help in the redesigning of a kitchen for the arthritic housewife and provide suitable aids, but prefers to suggest relevant commercially available equipment. Various voluntary organisations provide help for arthritic sufferers (see above).

Membership of the British Rheumatism and Arthritis Association is open to anyone concerned about the problems associated with rheumatism and arthritis, including sufferers. Their services include welfare facilities, holiday hotels and a wide selection of literature. There are 98 branches which members can attend for social evenings; outings and holiday trips are arranged. General services for the disabled, including the arthritic, are provided by the British Red Cross Society and the Central Council for the Care of the Disabled. An Aid Centre has been established by the Disabled Living Foundation at 346 Kensington High Street, London S.W.14 to provide an information service and a permanent exhibition of aids and equipment, which is primarily open for professional enquiries.

18
Prevention

Prevention of Certain Diseases
 Public health measures
 Control of infection
 Drug therapy
 Dietary measures
 Mechanical factors
Prevention of the Effects of Arthritic Diseases
Prevention of Symptoms
 Mechanical factors
 Emotional factors
 Weather
 Diet
 Occupation

With the strides that have been made in the understanding of rheumatic diseases a good deal can be done to prevent certain ones, to minimise the ill-effects of others, and to alleviate symptoms.

Prevention of Certain Diseases

Public health measures

These have been largely responsible for the dramatic drop in the incidence of rheumatic fever. Cramped and crowded households were responsible for epidemics of streptococcal sore throats. With the improvement in housing, the drop in the incidence of streptococcal infection has resulted in a sharp decline in the subsequent rheumatic fever which occurred in 1-5% of patients involved in these outbreaks of streptococcal infection.

Control of infection

Once a child has had an attack of rheumatic fever, the prophylactic use of penicillin or sulphonamides prevents the recurrence of streptococcal infections, and therefore of subsequent attacks of rheumatic fever. This is important in that further attacks of rheumatic fever are more likely to leave permanent damage to the heart valves. The control of venereal diseases will also obviate certain rheumatic complaints. Reiter's disease is the greatest hazard to which the promiscuous male is subject today. Any procedure involving injection of a joint should be conducted under conditions of strict asepsis, to avoid infection.

Drug therapy

Already we have noted that penicillin or sulphonamides will stop the streptococcal infections that trigger off rheumatic fever. In the case of gout, acute attacks can be prevented in the long term by lowering the level of serum uric acid, either by continuous treatment with drugs that excrete uric acid in the urine (uricosuric drugs such as probenecid, or sulphinpyrazone) or drugs that prevent the formation of uric acid (allopurinol). In a condition where there is great tissue breakdown, such as the treatment of leukaemia with cytotoxic drugs producing a marked rise in serum uric acid and the possibility of acute gout, allopurinol may be given prophylactically. Whilst serum uric acid is being mobilised from the body stores and excreted, acute attacks may develop. To prevent these colchicine is given three times a day.

Dietary measures

These may be important in gout. Although heredity is thought to be more important than alcohol consumption in this disease, there is evidence that alcohol plays a role in the development of attacks and sufferers should be advised to be moderate in their alcohol intake if not wholly abstemious.

The only other role in which diet is important is if the patient is overweight (Fig. 18.1). Where weightbearing joints are involved in any arthritic process, reduction of weight will reduce symptoms. Nature knows how best to teach us. The more we eat, the harder it is to get to the table!

Mechanical factors

These are important at times in producing disease and their avoidance can prevent arthritis. Treatment of congenital dislocation of the hip at birth has reduced the number of cases of osteoarthrosis of the hip from that cause. Other joint deformities may predispose to osteoarthrosis and the correction of position after a bad fracture may prevent degenerative joint disease. There is some evidence that osteoarthrosis is more prevalent in certain sportsmen, as discussed in the chapter on osteoarthrosis. This is probably related to injury, rather than the impacts occasioned by the sport.

It is important that injuries should be treated adequately and partially fit players not allowed to return to competitive sport, if subsequent osteoarthrosis is to be avoided. Likewise, certain work

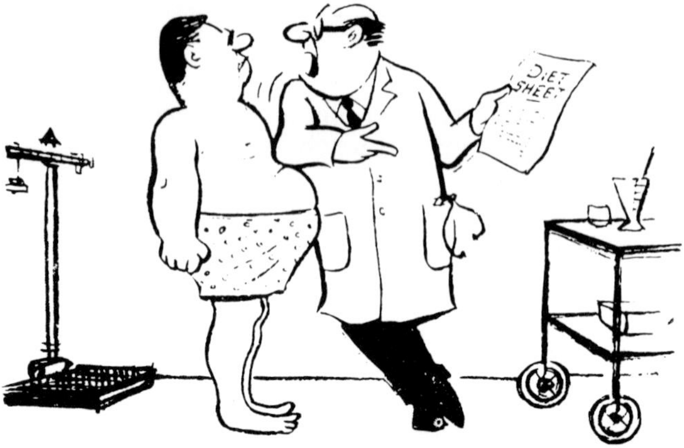

".......... *unless you are too fat*"

Fig. 18.1. The place of diet in prevention.

situations predispose to osteoarthrosis (Table 18.1). A change of job if symptoms of osteoarthrosis begin to appear may prevent further damage. Proper instructions in lifting will prevent back trouble, particularly in occupations such as nursing which involve lifting heavy objects or subjects (Fig. 18.2). The back is not a derrick and heavy objects should be lifted by placing the feet near the object, bending the knees and lifting with the back straight (Figs. 18.3 and 18.4). If twisting round, the feet should be moved and not the trunk twisted whilst carrying a heavy object.

Prevention of the Effects of Arthritic Diseases

The prevention of deformity is of prime importance in ankylosing spondylitis. This is discussed in Chapter 6.

The proper treatment of patients with rheumatoid arthritis will also help in the prevention of disabling deformities. No rheumatoid patients

Prevention

Osteoarthrosis — Occupational Factors
Underground roadway workers Miners Dockworkers Pneumatic drillers Cotton operatives Diamond cutters

Table 18.1

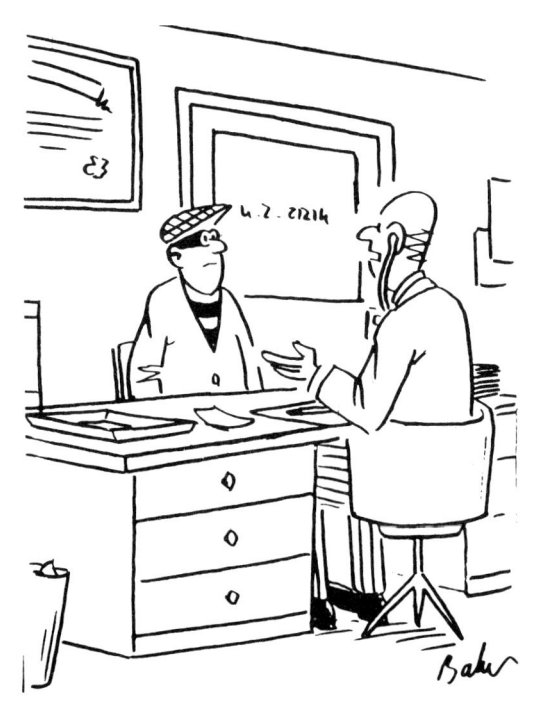

"Don't lift anything heavy.
Stick to small stuff such as jewellery."

Fig. 18.2. Proper instruction in lifting for sufferers from back complaints.

180 Rheumatism for Nurses & Remedial Therapists

Your back is not a derrick

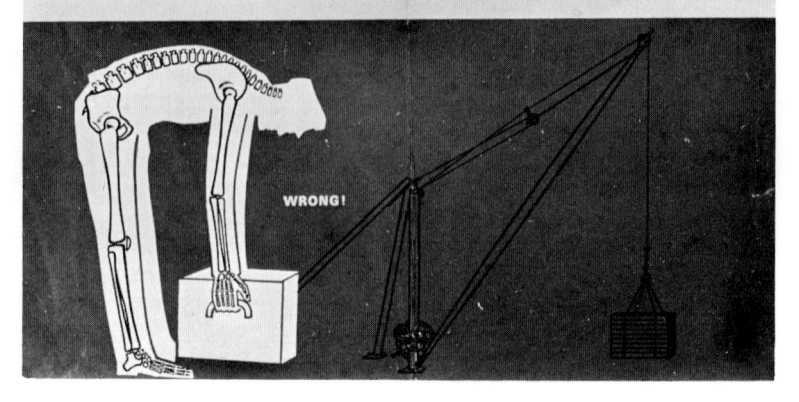

WRONG!

Fig. 18.3. Wrong way to lift.

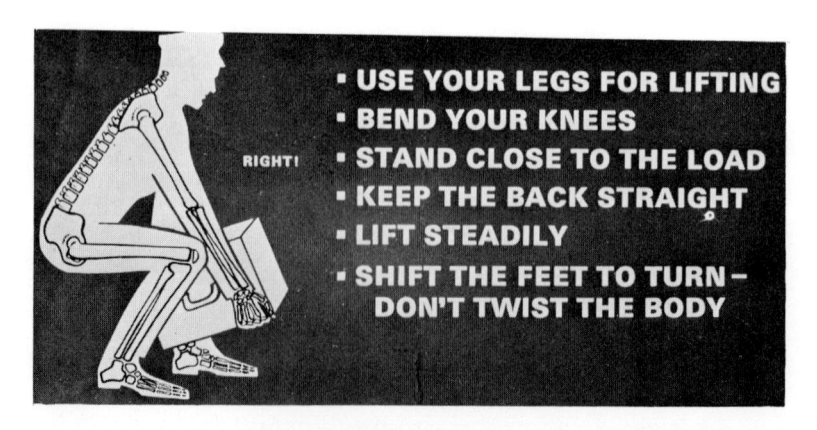

RIGHT!
- USE YOUR LEGS FOR LIFTING
- BEND YOUR KNEES
- STAND CLOSE TO THE LOAD
- KEEP THE BACK STRAIGHT
- LIFT STEADILY
- SHIFT THE FEET TO TURN – DON'T TWIST THE BODY

Fig. 18.4. Correct way to lift.

should be nursed with a pillow under their knees, lest a flexion deformity develops. Rest splints for knees, ankles, wrists and hands are beneficial (Chapter 16).

Prevention of Symptoms

Mechanical factors

Symptoms relating to the spine may be improved by attention to mechanical factors. Patients, especially middle-aged women, who experience pain from the cervical spine and around the shoulder girdle, should avoid carrying heavy shopping baskets, coal scuttles and other objects which drag down on the shoulder girdle. They should invest in a shopping basket on wheels and persuade their husband to lift the coal scuttle! Postural exercises to tone up the muscles around the shoulder girdle may also help to relieve symptoms.

For the sufferer from backache, a firm mattress or even a board under the mattress, may prevent pain.

Emotional factors

These may aggravate most rheumatic conditions. This is particularly true of pain round the shoulder girdle, and in certain circumstances may be the sole explanation of 'muscular rheumatism'. The avoidance of stressful situations may relieve pain, because tension is alleviated.

Weather

There is no evidence that climatic conditions cause any rheumatic diseases. However, cold and damp doubtless aggravate symptoms in many patients. A survey in Jamaica revealed a prevalence of rheumatic diseases similar to that in Great Britain, but the patients complained less.

Diet

Reducing weight may improve symptoms in lower limb joints. It is doubtful whether it prevents the actual disease, but symptomatically the benefit may be enormous. There is no evidence that the many quack diets which are advocated have any beneficial effect.

Occupation

The alteration of the working environment by a slight degree may produce a good deal of symptomatic benefit. Patients who have arthritis in the legs will be better with a sedentary job. Young men with ankylosing spondylitis are ill-advised to continue as garage mechanics, which involves contortion of the spine into difficult postures under unfavourable circumstances. A simple example of alteration in working conditions producing benefit is that of a 35-year-old man with rheumatoid arthritis, who was a patient of ours. He had marked involvement of the wrist. His job entailed hitting a button with his wrist hundreds of times a day. We visited the factory and with the co-operation of the management installed a lever which he could knock with his forearm, thus avoiding the need for hitting the button with his wrist. His symptoms were largely relieved, and as it happened production was speeded up! For heavy occupations like mining, if knees, hips or back are the site of severe symptoms, it may mean undertaking a surface job rather than continuing as a coal face worker.

19
Laboratory Investigations

Blood Tests
ESR
Haemoglobin level
White blood count
Platelet count
LE cells
Serum uric acid
Proteins
Calcium, phosphorus and alkaline phosphatase
Rheumatoid factor
Wasserman reaction
Brucella agglutinins
Anti-streptolysin O
Blood culture
Gonococcal complement fixation test

Urine Examination
Albumin
Pus cells
Sugar

Synovial Fluid
Organisms
Differential cell count
Crystals
Inflammatory and non-inflammatory effusions

Tissue Examination
Synovium
Nodule biopsy
Muscle biopsy
Lymph gland biopsy

Electrodiagnostic Tests
Electromyography
Nerve conduction studies

Radiology
Arthroscopy

A full clinical examination is necessary for the assessment of every rheumatic patient. In certain cases additional useful information may be gained from laboratory investigations and x-ray examination. These may be useful to help make a diagnosis, to assess the present activity of the disease, and to give an indication of the outlook for the patient.
  The areas of investigation are:
  1. Blood tests
  2. Urine examination
  3. Synovial fluid examination
  4. Tissue microscopy
  5. Electrodiagnostic tests
  6. X-ray examination
  7. Arthroscopy.

Blood Tests

Erythrocyte sedimentation rate

This is often abbreviated to ESR and sometimes to BSR (blood sedimentation rate). It measures the distance red and white cells settle in a column of blood in a capillary tube over a period of one hour. Normal values vary with age. As a rough guide figures of around 10 mm in the first hour in younger people and up to 20 or 25 mm in the first hour in older people are considered normal. Whenever there is any inflammation, from whatever cause, the ESR increases. It may be useful, therefore, in helping to differentiate arthritis which is inflammatory, such as rheumatoid arthritis or rheumatic fever, from that which is not inflammatory, such as osteoarthrosis or 'muscular rheumatism'.
  It may also help to determine the progress of disease. In patients with rheumatic fever, the joints may settle down but the heart may still be the site of active inflammation. One of the indications of this may be a raised ESR. Similarly, in active rheumatoid arthritis the ESR is raised roughly in proportion to the degree of active inflammation. However, in long standing disease, the sedimentation rate is sometimes raised without other evidence of inflammation in the joints.

Haemoglobin level (Hb)

Sometimes the haemoglobin is expressed in percentage terms, but more often these days it is expressed in g/dl. The normal haemoglobin is 14.2 g/dl in the blood, although women are often slightly below that. Patients with rheumatoid arthritis are frequently anaemic. This may be due to some blood loss from the drugs which the patient is receiving that have caused a small amount of bleeding from the stomach. (This is considered in Chapter 21.) Blood loss is not usually the important cause of the anaemia, and the red blood cells do not show the characteristic appearance resulting from blood loss. It may also be due to a suppression of the bone marrow manufacturing red blood cells due to the general disease. There is a slightly shortened life span of the red cells in this disease as well. Red cells in this condition are often somewhat pale (hypochromic), but usually of normal shape (normocytic). The level of haemoglobin is quite a good indication of the activity of the rheumatoid arthritis over a prolonged period, and as the disease abates so the haemoglobin rises. This may occur through natural remission of the arthritis, or it may be induced through drugs such as corticosteroids. In the latter case the haemoglobin may rise dramatically.

White blood count (W.b.c.)

The white blood count may be helpful in indicating infective arthritis. In that case there will be a considerable increase in white cells (leucocytosis). Occasionally this is seen in rheumatoid arthritis, but on the other hand a reduction in the number of white blood cells is sometimes seen (leucopaenia). Such a leucopaenia is more frequently seen with systemic lupus erythematosus, or with Felty's syndrome in which there is a large spleen and rheumatoid arthritis. Occasionally the drugs which the patient is receiving may stop the manufacture of blood, giving either a complete shutdown of blood formation (aplastic anaemia) or a failure to form polymorphonuclear white blood cells (agranulocytosis).

Platelet count

Some drugs which patients with rheumatic diseases are given suppress the formation of platelets (thrombocytopaenia). Gold and penicillamine are examples of such compounds. The patient may develop small pin point areas of bleeding in the skin (purpura). If this happens they should be admitted to hospital immediately. A subarachnoid haemorrhage can occur, since bleeds can occur throughout the body.

LE cells

In systemic lupus erythematosus the blood can be made to form typical LE cells (Fig. 19.1). These tests are done less frequently these days, and antinuclear factor is more often sought in the serum by an immunological method.

Serum uric acid

In gout serum uric acid is elevated and it is a useful diagnostic pointer. However, the only completely diagnostic test for acute gout is to aspirate urate crystals from the affected joint. It must be remembered, however, that other things, apart from primary gout, will raise the serum uric acid. If the excretion of serum uric acid is hindered by kidney disease or by small doses of aspirin, a raised level of serum uric

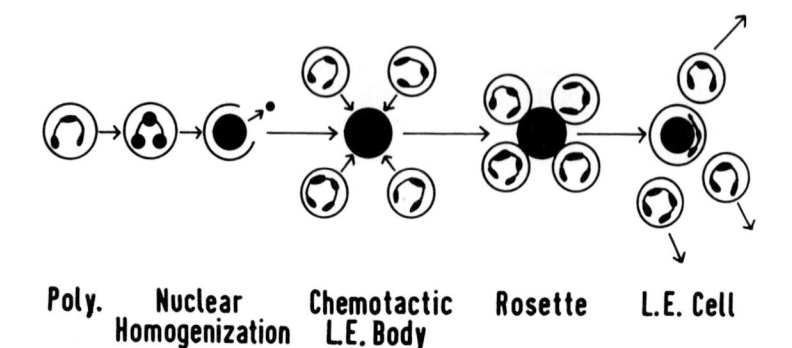

Fig. 19.1. Stages in the development of LE cell diagrammatically.

acid can be produced. Similarly, it may be raised if uric acid is produced in excess, as in leukaemia due to the excessive destruction of white cells, or in polycythaemia where excessive red blood cells are broken down. Relatives of gouty patients may also have a raised serum uric acid without symptoms of gout. The uric acid level may have been artificially lowered because of a drug the patient is receiving, such as those designed to excrete uric acid through the kidney (uricosuric agents). The patient may also be on a drug such as allopurinol which blocks the formation of uric acid. Indeed the level of serum uric acid may be used to monitor the effectiveness of these drugs in the long term management of gout.

Proteins

Both the total level of protein in the blood, and the level of the individual protein fractions must be considered, as compensating abnormalities in separate fractions may make the total blood level normal. This is often so in rheumatoid arthritis, where the level of globulin may be high, while that of albumin may be low. If there is a severe derangement of the protein pattern, one may think of a complication of rheumatoid disease (such as amyloidosis), a more diffuse disorder of connective tissue, or a rather unusual disease of the elderly, multiple myelomatosis.

Calcium, phosphorus and alkaline phosphatase

In certain bone diseases such as osteomalacia (an adult form of rickets), the calcium may be low and the alkaline phosphatase raised. Paget's disease, which is quite frequently seen in the elderly, may give a very elevated alkaline phosphatase. Disorders of the parathyroid gland may also produce rheumatic complaints and may be picked up by their effect on the level of calcium and phosphorus.

Rheumatoid factor

In rheumatoid arthritis 80% of patients have an abnormal protein, called rheumatoid factor, in their blood which clumps together (agglutinates) specially coated sheep red cells. This is called the sheep cell agglutination test (SCAT) or the differential agglutination test (DAT). It is useful in diagnosis. The absence of rheumatoid factor may also alert the physician to the possibility of other diagnoses, such as Reiter's disease, and the arthritis associated with various bowel disorders, or with psoriasis. It has also been noticed that where rheumatoid factor is absent from the serum of patients who apparently have rheumatoid arthritis, their outlook is better. Higher concentrations are associated with a poorer prognosis and a greater liability to develop the systemic complications of rheumatoid disease. A similar test may be used with latex particles specially coated. This is known as the latex fixation test.

Wasserman reaction (WR)

This is positive in syphilis. Tertiary syphilis is rarely seen these days, but systemic lupus erythematosus may be associated with a positive WR. This is termed a 'biological false positive' test for syphilis.

Brucella agglutinins

These may be sought where brucellosis is suspected. This may give a vague type of arthritis and affects the spine and peripheral joints. The patient may have a fever and may present with a pyrexia of unknown origin.

Anti-streptolysin O (ASO)

This is an antibody to a product of streptococci. The titre of anti-streptolysin O may be raised in patients with rheumatic fever. Rheumatic fever follows a streptococcal sore throat in only 1-5% of patients so the raised titre does not necessarily indicate the diagnosis of rheumatic fever—it only means the patient has had a streptococcal infection.

Blood culture

Sometimes organisms circulate and grow in the blood (septicaemia). Patients with rheumatoid arthritis are liable to get an infected joint and sometimes a septicaemia develops from this. It may also happen in osteomyelitis, where the bone is infected, usually with staphylococcus aureus. Again it is carefully sought in patients with long-standing rheumatic heart disease in whom it is feared infection has developed on the valve producing sub-acute bacterial endocarditis.

Gonococcal complement fixation test (GCFT)

This used to be done where gonococcal arthritis was suspected. The test, however, is notoriously inaccurate, and positive results may be obtained when the patient has no evidence of past or present gonorrhoea.

Urine Examination

Urine should be tested at the initial examination of any patient with a rheumatic disorder.

Albumin

In patients on certain drugs, such as gold or penicillamine, it should be tested routinely for albumin (albuminuria). When gold is being given, albuminuria should be sought before each injection is given. Albuminuria may also occur as a result of a direct involvement of the kidney from rheumatic diseases such as systemic lupus erythematosus, polyarteritis nodosa, and amyloidosis complicating conditions such as rheumatoid arthritis.

Pus cells

These may be sought where urinary infection is suspected. In Reiter's disease they are sometimes found in the first specimen in the morning.

Laboratory Investigations

Sugar (glycosuria)

Sugar should be sought where the patient is taking corticosteroids, since these may unmask a latent diabetes mellitus.

Synovial Fluid

In normal joints synovial fluid is present in very small quantities (0.5 ml in a knee joint). It is very sticky and has a crystal clear, yellow appearance. In rheumatoid arthritis it is often markedly increased in amount, so that aspirations of over 100 ml are sometimes made. The fluid is thin and cloudy. In osteoarthrosis there may also be an increase in the amount of joint fluid, although not to such a marked extent as in rheumatoid arthritis. The fluid is stickier than rheumatoid fluid and is golden yellow, crystal clear in appearance. Aspiration of a joint is frequently done for diagnostic purposes. The procedure is described in Chapter 20. In certain circumstances, such as a Baker's cyst behind the knee in the popliteal fossa or even tracking down into the calf, the fluid may be very thick with large flakes of fibrin. In that case a much larger needle will be required.

Organisms

Where a pyogenic arthritis is suspected, either in its own right or superimposed upon rheumatoid inflammation of the joint, aspiration is essential to make a diagnosis and institute proper treatment. Fluid is immediately smeared and stained with Gram stain to detect bacteria, and then cultured. If organisms grow, their sensitivity to various antibiotics is tested.

If tuberculosis is suspected joint fluid may also be aspirated for diagnostic purposes. It is smeared and stained with a special stain (Ziehl-Neilsen) to display 'acid fast bacilli'. Indeed tuberculosis is sometimes called 'acid fast disease', especially when talking before the patient lest they should be unduly alarmed. The fluid in this case has to be cultured for a much longer time, and guinea pig inoculation is performed before a diagnosis can be excluded.

Differential cell count

One portion of the fluid is taken into an anticoagulant and a cell count done. There are few cells in normal synovial fluid, but in a pyogenic arthritis there may be over 20,000 polymorphonuclear leucocytes per cubic millimetre. In a tuberculous effusion the white blood cells will be mainly lymphocytes, which have a single, dark staining, central nucleus which largely fills the cell. Rheumatoid effusions often have a large number of polymorphonuclear leucocytes, and these may be reported as 'pus cells'. Although they are the same as the pus cells one gets in an infective arthritis, it must not be thought that they necessarily indicate infection. They are just the manifestation of an acute inflammatory reaction.

Crystals

Crystals of uric acid may be found in gout. These show up in a particular way with a special microscope (the polarising microscope). There is another condition called pseudo-gout in which calcium pyrophosphate crystals are seen. Whereas uric acid crystals are needle shaped, those of calcium pyrophosphate are rhomboidal (Fig. 12.4).

Inflammatory and non-inflammatory effusions

Examination of the joint fluid may be useful in distinguishing inflammatory from non-inflammatory (usually osteoarthrotic) effusions. In inflammatory effusions there are many white cells, chiefly polymorphonuclear leucocytes. As the effusion becomes subacute or chronic, however, there may be more mononuclear (single nucleus) cells and cholesterol crystals may appear. The protein content of the fluid is high in an inflammatory arthritis, and the sugar level may be low. Rheumatoid factor, which is present in the serum, may also be present in the joint fluid in rheumatoid arthritis—and occasionally it has been reported in the joint fluid when it is absent from the serum.

There is a special test sometimes done on joint fluid which consists of adding acetic acid. In normal and osteoarthrotic fluid this produces a tight mass of precipitated material. In rheumatoid arthritis, however, the clot is stringy. This is called the mucin clot test.

Tissue Examination

Synovium

A piece of the synovial membrane may be examined under the microscope. This is obtained either by an open operation under general anaesthetic, by a special biopsy needle (percutaneous biopsy) under local anaesthetic, or by viewing the inside of the joint with an arthroscope and selecting the tissue to be removed.

Synovial biopsy may be of value in diagnosing pyogenic arthritis, tuberculous arthritis and gout. It may also be helpful in distinguishing osteoarthrosis from rheumatoid arthritis.

Laboratory Investigations

Where a single joint is involved, biopsy is frequently done to exclude the possibility of tuberculosis. That apart, biopsy of the synovial membrane is often not of great value. Occasionally tumour may be picked up or some rare kind of joint infection.

Nodule biopsy

This may be helpful. The appearance in rheumatoid arthritis is distinctive. In gout a deposit of urate forms a tophus. This may show as a nodule in an olecranon bursa, on the hands, or in the pinna of the ear.

Muscle biopsy

In diffuse disorders of connective tissue such as polyarteritis nodosa or dermatomyositis, a muscle biopsy may enable a diagnosis to be made. These diagnoses are important from the point of view of treatment and frequently require further confirmation by muscle biopsy. Sometimes this is done under local anaesthetic, and rather more commonly under a general anaesthetic. In rheumatoid arthritis muscle wasting may be associated with peripheral nerve changes or with wasting associated with disuse. Muscle biopsy may be undertaken to differentiate these.

Lymph gland biopsy

This is sometimes undertaken to help in the diagnosis of a rheumatic disorder. However, it is frequently confusing in a disease like rheumatoid arthritis, where the lymph glands are commonly enlarged. Their appearance under the microscope often simulates other diseases such as Hodgkin's disease. If an underlying cancer is suspected, or a disease such as sacroidosis, then gland biopsy may be of help.

Electrodiagnostic Tests

Electromyography

During activity of a muscle it gives off an electrical discharge which produces a characteristic pattern on the oscilloscope, or the signal can be translated into sound. If there are problems with nerves, different patterns of impulse are picked up at rest and activity. Primary problems with muscles also produce some alteration of the electrical pattern.

Nerve conduction studies

If a nerve is compressed, for example the median nerve in the carpal tunnel, this produces a slowing of the rate of the electrical impulse along its path. These nerve conduction times can be measured and the site of entrapment of the nerve localised.

Radiology

X-ray of the joints may give some diagnostic clues about rheumatoid arthritis, osteoarthrosis or gout. In rheumatoid arthritis (Fig. 3.8) there may be thinning of the bones adjacent to the joint margins (juxta-articular osteoporosis), soft tissue swelling, loss of joint space due to destruction of the cartilage, and erosive changes beginning at the margin of the joint. Later, deformity and even disorganisation of the joint may occur.

In osteoarthrosis (Chapter 4) osteophytes are present at the margin of the joint; there may be loss of joint space due to the flaking away of the cartilage, thickening of the adjacent bone (eburnation), and cystic changes in the underlying bone. In gout the characteristic features are punched out areas or cystic changes, due to the deposition of urate (Fig. 12.5a).

X-rays may also be useful in ascertaining the presence of a fracture. Sometimes a patient is sent up to a Rheumatic Clinic with a diagnosis of arthritis of a joint, whereas in fact they have sustained a fracture in the region of it. A tuberculous arthritis may show calcification around the joint. If infective arthritis is untreated there will be considerable destruction of the joint progressing rapidly. Paget's disease is frequently picked up on x-ray of bones. It commonly affects the pelvis, the femur or the tibia. This may or may not produce symptoms. Radio-opaque dye may be injected into the joint to outline it—this is called arthrography. It is particularly useful in the knee, where a posterior outpouching of the synovial membrane into the popliteal fossa (Baker's cyst) may track down into the calf and simulate a deep vein thrombosis if it ruptures. The technique is also used in the shoulder and wrist. X-rays of other regions may help to establish a diagnosis. For instance a chest x-ray may show a cancer of the lung, from which deposits have spread to bones.

Barium studies of the gastrointestinal tract (barium meal and follow through, or barium enema) may show the presence of Crohn's disease, ulcerative colitis, or a peptic ulcer. The last is not directly related to any rheumatic condition, but is very important because so much of the therapy given for rheumatic conditions is liable to produce or aggravate any ulcer. It is important, therefore, that if a patient does have indigestion that the presence of an ulcer should be realised.

Arthroscopy

The arthroscope is an instrument similar to a small cystoscope which can be inserted into the knee joint allowing a direct view of the inside of the joint. This technique is probably of greatest value in the diagnosis of internal derangements of the knee. The menisci, cruciate ligaments and articular surfaces can all be inspected. The diagnosis of chondromalacia patellae can also be made by direct observation. Rheumatologists make greatest use of the arthroscope to inspect the inflamed synovium and to take biopsies of the most severely affected piece of synovium for diagnostic purposes. The procedure is described in Chapter 20.

20
Nursing Care

General Care
Diet
Alleviation of Pain
Prevention of Deformity
Nursing Observation
Patient's Morale
Rehabilitation
Special Procedures
Community Care
Health Visitor

Too often the nursing care of the arthritic patient has been envisaged in terms of treatment of the patient with rheumatic fever at the turn of the century. A patient with acutely inflamed joints is packed in cotton wool, kept carefully covered by warm blankets and maintained at complete bed rest in a darkened, secluded corner of the ward. Today rheumatic fever in this country is mercifully rare and more dynamic concepts govern therapy.

The nursing care required by any patients who suffers from a rheumatic disease may be based on the following principles:
1. The general care and comfort of the patient. In nearly all the conditions that have been described in previous chapters, there is a constitutional disease allied to the arthritis. There are acute phases when the patient is extremely ill and less acute phases.
2. The alleviation of pain. Pain is present to some degree in most cases.
3. The prevention of deformity.
4. Careful observation.
5. The support and encouragement of the patient and the maintenance of morale.
6. The rehabilitation of the patient.
7. Special procedures.

The nurse plays her part not only during the acute phase of the disease when hospital admission is required, but also in the out-patient clinics and the patient's home. Throughout she is a member of a team comprising among others, doctors both in and out of hospital, physiotherapists, occupational therapists, social workers, chiropodists and members of voluntary organisations. While many of the aspects of nursing described here are especially applicable to hospital care, the principles involved are just as important in the patient's home.

General Care

In the actue phase, the patient with arthritis is nursed at rest. The bed should have a firm mattress and fracture boards may be put under the mattress if there is a tendency for the mattress to sag. This is particularly necessary if there are back problems. The patient must have sufficient pillows and be well supported for comfort. A bed cradle will keep the weight of the bed clothes off tender, inflamed joints of the lower limb, but a thin flanelette sheet next to the patient and underneath the cradle will ensure warmth. The ill-effects of bed rest must not be forgotten, the development of contractures, the wasting of muscles, clotting in the leg veins and subsequent pulmonary embolus, thinning of the bones (osteoporosis), renal calculus, infection in the lungs and pressure sores.

Clothing should be light, warm and easily put on. As much movement in this acute phase can produce pain, the nurse must handle the limbs carefully, supporting each fully so that undue and painful movement does not occur. Lifting and turning the patient must also be done slowly and carefully; any jarring of joints must be avoided. The limbs should be placed in a position as near the position of function as possible and splints may be used to ensure this—preventing pain and undue deformity. Another patient who requires particularly careful handling is the rheumatoid on long-term corticosteroids, since the skin is often fragile. Abrasions from knocking against sharp corners can readily develop into chronic ulcers. The skin over the shins may be so thin that shin guards of plastazote may be indicated.

Another patient who requires careful handling is the rheumatoid with cervical spine involvement. The danger of subluxation in this region is that pressure may be placed on the spinal cord, and a paraplegia or tetraplegia develop.

As the patient in the acute phase often has some degree of pyrexia, and is frequently given drugs which encourage sweating, a daily blanket bath is essential. The patient who is sweating profusely will require additional washing to remove sweat. In these patients, great care must be taken to make sure that skin folds are thoroughly dried and a little dusting powder applied between to prevent soreness. It is particularly important to see that the buttocks and natal cleft are kept clean and dry, to prevent the formation of small blisters which can lead to the development of a sore. All other care, including change of position, must be taken to prevent skin breaks.

Oedema of the legs may develop due to inactivity, the poor muscle tone of the legs, the sluggish venous return in varicose veins (which are commoner in patients with osteoarthrosis than in other hospital patients), pressure from swollen knees or alongside inflamed joints. It may be relieved by elevation of the end of the bed at nights. In severer cases postural drainage of the legs in the morning may be needed. The legs are elevated on a frame (like half a deckchair) for half an hour, and then a Bisgaard blue-line bandage is applied for the rest of the day. The elevation is repeated and the bandages are re-applied in the evening. Often this suffices to get rid of the fluid. These efforts may be supplemented in the physiotherapy department by faradism under pressure, and elastic stockings may be required as a long term measure. It should not be forgotten, however, that arthritic patients often have great difficulty in pulling on elastic stockings.

Diet

This is not a problem with arthritis patients as far as special provision is concerned. Those with gout should have a low purine diet and avoid excess alcohol. Obese patients with damage to weightbearing joints should reduce weight. Apart from these considerations, a well balanced, nutritious diet is all that is required. Rheumatoid patients are often underweight, partly due to the systemic effect of the disease, partly to loss of appetite from disease and drugs, and partly to difficulty in making meals. A dietary survey we undertook showed they had an inadequate intake of many things such as vitamin D and calcium. Fad diets are to be deprecated—there is no evidence that they have any curative or beneficial effects.

Alleviation of Pain

Rest relieves pain in many cases. This is why a period of bed rest for patients with acute rheumatoid arthritis, with osteoarthrosis of weight-bearing joints, or with prolapsed intervertebral disc may be so beneficial. The patient with chronic joint damage also benefits from an hour's rest on the bed after lunch, the joints being put in a good position.

The place of plasters for resting the joints is discussed in Chapter 17. When plaster splints are applied the nurse must be particularly careful. Any signs of the plaster being too tight, such as colour changes of the limb distal to the plaster, swelling or pain, should be reported immediately. If the plaster is too tight, it will require removal. Rubbing over a bony prominence or at the edge of the plaster must also be avoided lest abrasion of the skin occurs. It may require a new plaster, although at other times the insertion of a small piece of sponge rubber, or dampening the edge and remoulding it, or cutting off some of the plaster may suffice. Occasionally pressure over the region of the head of the fibula produces a common peroneal (lateral popliteal) nerve palsy with foot drop, and this should be reported immediately. Drugs will be administered to relieve pain and the nurse will note whether these drugs have the desired effect.

Prevention of Deformity

The patient requires a firm mattress and the limbs must be placed gently into a good position. To ensure this spints may be used for the limbs—sometimes these are worn continuously, but often they are worn at night only. These splints are usually made from plaster of Paris, but may be made from polythene or plastazote and are tailored to fit the individual patient. The nurses are responsible for the actual application of the splints and care must be taken to see that the skin is absolutely dry before they are fastened in position. Undue pain or soreness associated with the splint must be noticed and reported. Velcro straps are used so that when the patient has to put the splints on herself she can manage, since buckles are usually too difficult for a patient with a rheumatoid hand to manage. Bad positioning in bed may produce deformity and must be avoided, although the patient may temporarily feel more comfortable in these positions (Figs. 20.1 and 20.2).

One reason for treating patients with early acute rheumatoid arthritis in hospital is to familiarise them with the discipline of rest splints at night. To prevent foot drop a foot board may be placed across the cradle at right angles to the bed.

If the patient has such fragile skin that splints cannot be tolerated, proper positioning of the legs may be obtained by sponge rubber supports.

A flexion deformity of an osteoarthrotic hip may be overcome by periods of lying prone.

Nursing Observation

The patient in the acute phase of arthritis requires careful observation. Temperature, pulse and respirations will be taken and recorded four-hourly.

Increased pain and tenderness or involvement of other joints will be noticed whilst attending to the patient's needs and reported.

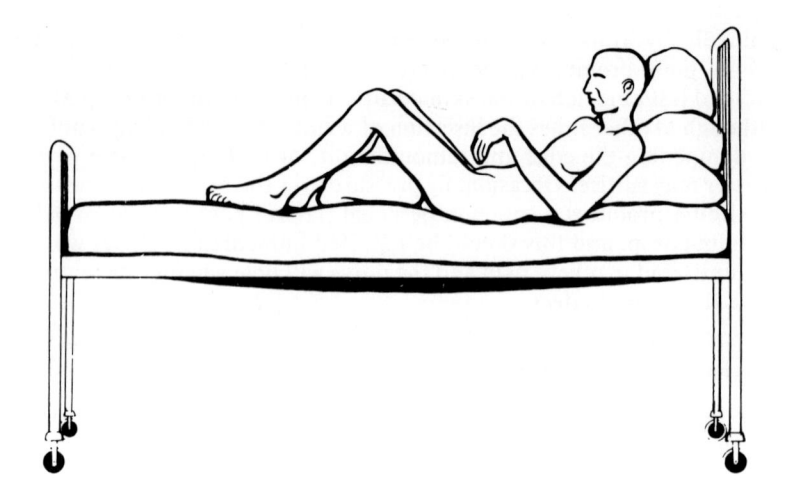

Fig. 20.1. Bad positioning in bed.

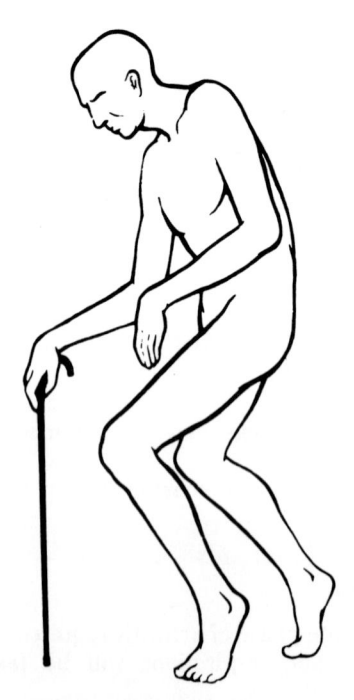

Fig. 20.2. Deformities from bad positioning in bed.

The nurse is in a particularly good position to observe the patients first thing in the morning when their capabilities are at their lowest. A patient whose hands are quite free by mid-morning may be unable to work on waking and may struggle with breakfast, but these activities are rarely seen by the doctor who may wish to prescribe appropriate medication to overcome this problem. It is the nurse's responsibility to administer any drugs prescribed by the physician and these are discussed in Chapter 21. Accurate timing of drug administration is important if sustained effects are to be achieved with short acting drugs. This may mean departure from the traditional 'medicine round' times. As more is known about drug interaction within the patient's gut it is likely that drugs will have to be given at more precise intervals than is the custom at present. Analgesics are often given as a supplement to the antirheumatic medication as needed (i.e. a p.r.n. basis). It is important that these drugs are not unnecessarily withheld to fall in with 'medicine round' time.

Equally it is the nurse's responsibility to report on the effectiveness of these drugs or any untoward effect which they may produce. If pain at night keeps the patient awake, or morning stiffness is a pronounced feature, this should be drawn to the physician's attention, with the possibility of re-timing the doses or altering the drug regime.

Urine testing is of particular importance when gold or penicillamine are given. Albuminuria is a contra-indication to the use of either drug. Its development may also be due to a complication of the disease, such as amyloidosis in rheumatoid arthritis, or renal involvement in systemic lupus erythematosus or polyarteritis nodosa. Glycosuria may develop if steroids are taken.

Patient's Morale

Often patients wiil share their underlying anxieties about the disease and its implications with the nursing staff. In association with the physician reassurance may be a powerful factor in treatment. The patient may have an unjustifiable fear that she is going to become crippled and that there is no real hope for her condition. Moreover, anxiety about the family and about the home may dominate the patient's outlook. The help of the medical social worker may relieve the situation.

Rehabilitation

After a period of immobility the patient may require help in establishing a proper walking pattern. The nurse may work in collaboration with the physiotherapist on teaching the patient to take even steps. The ability to turn round may have been lost also, and the patient will need to be taught the placing of the feet and of a walking stick, if this is required, during this manoeuvre.

Following initial bed rest graded activity is usually prescribed. The nurse should encourage the patients to do their periods of exercise without supervision (e.g. quadriceps exercises and hand exercises).

Special Procedures

In addition to the normal day-to-day care of the patient, the nurse will perform or assist with a number of procedures. These include some of general application, such as dressing of ulcers, post-operative care of wounds and removal of stitches. Some routine procedures such as collection of mid-stream urine specimens or catheterisation of female patients may be made more difficult by the restriction of joint movement in hips and knees. Both subcutaneous injections of ACTH and intramuscular injections of gold or iron may be given. Both these require special precautions. Injection of gold must be preceded by a urine test for albumin and an enquiry of the patient regarding rash, itch or sore throat. Iron injections must be given using the Z-track technique, otherwise tattooing (staining) of the skin surface may occur because iron has oozed back along the needle track (Fig. 21.1).

Intra-lesional injections of corticosteroid may be used in patients with such conditions as tennis elbow, tenosynovitis or carpal tunnel syndrome. The nurse will be required to assist in the same way as when joints are aspirated or injected.

Aspiration of joints may be undertaken for diagnostic or therapeutic purposes. After appropriate scrubbing or sterile hand preparation, the doctor will clean the skin over the joint to be entered. Local anaesthetic is usually used, with infiltration from skin to synovium. An aspiration needle is then inserted and fluid removed. This should be collected in a sterile container for culture and other appropriate investigations. At this stage local corticosteroid may be injected. This must be of the type labelled 'for intra-articular use'. Plain hydrocortisone is unacceptable. The needle is then removed and a plaster put over the puncture site. This should be left in place for two days. If a weightbearing joint has been injected the patient must rest for two days in order to prevent the occurrence of destructive 'steroid arthropathy'.

A similar procedure is used for injection of radio-active isotopes such as gold or yttrium. The joint is punctured and may be aspirated. The isotope, diluted in saline, is then injected and a 'flush' of 10 mls saline is then injected to clear isotope from the needle and prevent radiation burns in the needle track. The injected limb is immobilised for three days after injection to prevent spread of radio-active material from the joint. No hazard exists to staff or other patients and no special precautions are required for disposal of the patients urine or faeces. Arthroscopy is being increasingly used for viewing the inside of joints, usually the knee, and obtaining biopsies under direct vision. This procedure is carried out in the operating theatre under general or local anaesthetic. Normal theatre procedure is used for preparation and draping of the limb. The knee is aspirated and re-distended with saline either by direct intra-articular injection or by a drip inserted into the knee which runs throughout the procedure. The arthroscope is an instrument like a miniature cystoscope. It is inserted in the same way as an aspiration needle and the joint viewed, photographed and biopsied through it. The limb may be wrapped in wool post-operatively, and may be swollen for a couple of days. Re-educative physiotherapy, with particular stress on quadriceps exercises, should be undertaken from the first post-operative day.

Community Care

The District Nurse may help in the recognition of side effects of drugs and may also help to check the correct dosage. Advice may be given on whether the diet is adequate, or whether help is needed with a reducing diet. She may also need to undertake dressings where the skin has broken down, or after surgery. Where injections are prescribed, and the patient or a relative cannot undertake these, the District Nurse may be required to give them. Gold injections are given intra-muscularly at intervals of one week to one month. The urine should be checked for albumin before administering the dose and not given if albuminuria is present, nor if the patient complains of itching or a rash. ACTH is given by subcutaneous injections—usually in a long-acting form two or three times a week. Arthritic patients are often anaemic and intra-muscular injections of iron are sometimes prescribed—usually to a total of 1 gram.

Where the arthritic patient is bedfast she will need to be nursed in a light, sufficiently heated, cheerful room. If possible the bed should be near a window, allowing the patient to have a view of the world outside. She should be encouraged with tempting meals, and depression avoided by endeavouring to maintain her interests, e.g. radio, reading, television and visitors. Mobility should be encouraged where the conditions allow this. Particular care must be taken with pressure areas and real or artificial sheepskins are of great value to the wasted arthritic patient. Bed cradles may be required to relieve the weight of the bed clothes. Examination of the skin should be made for infection and general nursing care will be given. Personal hygiene in this respect is important and the maintenance of morale imperative.

Health Visitor

The Health Visitor is another member of the nursing profession who performs a vital function in this context. She bridges the gap between home and hospital. The ideal situation is where the Health Visitor is attached to the hospital Department and visits handicapped arthritic patients after discharge. In Leeds we have been particularly fortunate in having two Health Visitors attached to a Rehabilitation Unit of the hospital. Their work has been described in Chapter 17 when rehabilitation was discussed in detail. In this situation a planned programme of after care can be organised in conjunction with the community services and the patient's general practitioner. The Health Visitor reinforces the advice given in hospital particularly with regard to drugs, and she may liaise with the physiotherapy and occupational therapy departments after the patient has been discharged. Assessment needs to be made of the home conditions and attitudes of the patient, and of active help which is available. The Health Visitor and the Medical Social Worker will then mobilise domiciliary services according to the individual patient's needs (e.g. home helps, meals on wheels, voluntary help with shopping and social visiting of the lonely).

The Health Visitor has a supportive role in times of stress, sometimes acting as a therapeutic listener, or in some instances referring patients to agencies best able to cope with their particular problems. These may include the housing department as far as rehousing on medical grounds is concerned, or major home adaptation such as widening the doors for wheelchairs. Arthritis, like any other handicap, puts a strain on the marriage relationship and help may be needed from marriage guidance counsellors, advice on family planning or sexual problems from Family Planning Clinics or their domiciliary services, and help in caring for children (such as play groups, nursery schools, day nurseries and child minders). The breakdown of marriage is not uncommon among these patients and they may require free legal aid in the case of divorce and much support during this period.

The strain of coping with a handicapped person may be too great at times. It is essential to recognise early signs of breakdown in patients or relatives, so that relief can be given and crisis situations avoided. With the aid of the patient's general practitioner it may be possible to negotiate with the consultant physician to have the patient back for two or three weeks to give the relatives a break from caring, and fortify them ready to carry on when the patient returns home.

Some teaching may be required as regards suitable diets, so that the immobilised arthritic does not put on too much weight. Prevention of accidents due to loose stair rods, small mats or inadequate lighting is important, as is the rearrangement of furniture to facilitate a wheelchair. It is vital that arthritics should realise that they are still wanted and can be useful members of society. To this end liaison with government rehabilitation units, employment agencies and social services about sheltered workshops may be required. Keeping the handicapped patient interested and stimulated is one of the hardest tasks for the relatives and community workers. Liaison with charitable organisations such as the British Rheumatism Association, which gives help by providing radios, televisions, monthly social meetings, and transport for the housebound, may be invaluable. There is a great need for reassurance during visits, and help for patients and relatives with problems. Adapting to new situations, emotional adjustments, financial worries, together with housing difficulties and learning to accept permanent disabilities, are the hardest parts the arthritic has to bear. Many patients have months before they go outside their homes. It is not only their difficulty in walking but a dislike of the neighbours looking at them that is a trial. Patients need reassurance and encouragement at each visit in order that they may achieve their fullest possible mobility.

21
Drug Therapy in Rheumatic Diseases

Analgesic Drugs
  Paracetamol
  Phenacetin
  Dextropropoxyphene
  Codeine
  Dihydrocodeine
  Pentazocine
  Pethidine, morphine and other opiates

Analgesic/Anti-inflammatory Drugs
  Salicylates
    Side effects
    Salicylate preparations
  Phenylbutazone
    Side effects
  Indomethacin
    Side effects
  Fenamates
  Benorylate
  Propionic acid derivatives
    Ibuprofen
    Fenoprofen
    Ketoprofen
    Naproxen
  Azapropazone

Anti-inflammatory Drugs
  Corticosteroids
    Side effects
    Corticosteroid preparations
    Intra-articular corticosteroids
  Gold
    Side effects
  Antimalarial drugs

Muscle Relaxants
Psychiatric Drugs
Haematinics
New Forms of Therapy

D-penicillamine
Immunosuppressive drugs
Glossary of Drugs

The most frequent symptom in the rheumatic diseases is pain. This may be caused, or accompanied, by inflammation. Muscle spasm is frequently produced by joint pain, and prolonged painful conditions almost invariably give rise to psychological strain in the patients. The majority of the drugs used in the treatment of rheumatic diseases are directed against one or more of these symptoms.

Primary targets	*Secondary targets*
Pain	Muscle spasm
Inflammation	Psychological stress

Chart 1 Targets of Drugs used in the Treatment of Rheumatic Diseases.

In addition some other groups of drugs are used to combat more specific problems, often involving one particular disease process. The best example is the use of drugs which decrease the production or increase the excretion of uric acid in patients with gout. Anaemia is often a problem in patients with rheumatoid arthritis and will require appropriate therapy, and the poor diet taken by many rheumatic patients may require vitamin supplements.

Analgesic Drugs

Analgesics are drugs which act to reduce pain either by a local effect on the sensory nerves or a central effect on the centres in the brain concerned with the appreciation of pain. Their place in rheumatology is limited, as the combination of an anti-inflammatory effect, found in the more widely used analgesic/anti-inflammatory drugs, is usually desirable if pain relief is to be adequate.

Paracetamol

This is the most widely used of the analgesic drugs. It is available as a variety of proprietary brands, all of which contain 0.5 g paracetamol. It is also marketed in a soluble form and in combination with other mild analgesics such as codeine. In general, the use of such combinations is undesirable. Paracetamol is a mild analgesic which has the great advantage that it is less likely to cause gastric upset than aspirin. Patients with rheumatic diseases tend to need large doses ranging from 1 g to 2 g three to four times daily. Even in these doses the degree of analgesia is often inadequate.

Paracetamol

Advantages	*Disadvantages*
Well tolerated	Mild analgesic—often inadequate
Does not cause gastric bleeding	

Chart 2

Side effects are mainly of gastro-intestinal upset although this is not accompanied by bleeding.

Phenacetin

Paracetamol is a metabolite of phenacetin, which has been incriminated in causing a severe type of renal damage called analgesic nephropathy. There is as yet no convincing evidence that paracetamol causes similar damage.

Phenacetin

Advantages	*Disadvantages*
None	IMPLICATED IN CAUSING ANALGESIC NEPHROPATHY SHOULD NOT BE USED

Chart 3

Because of analgesic nephropathy, phenacetin has been withdrawn from many preparations which formerly contained it and its use has been confined to prescription drugs only by the Medicines (Phenacetin Prohibition) Order, 1974. Phenacetin-containing analgesics should not be used in the treatment of rheumatic diseases.

Dextropropoxyphene

This is a mild analgesic which is rarely used alone. The combination of dextropropoxyphene and paracetamol is claimed to show synergism, that is the effect of giving the two drugs together is greater than would be expected from their individual potencies. This combination is quite widely used where paracetamol alone is inadequate. Side effects of dextropropoxyphene include indigestion, dizziness, light-headedness and nausea.

Dextropropoxyphene	
Advantages	Disadvantages
Possible synergistic effect with paracetamol	Not very effective alone.
Generally well tolerated	Side effects, when they occur, may be disturbing to the patient

Chart 4

Codeine

Codeine is an analgesic of moderate potency which is rarely used alone because of its liability to cause constipation. It appears in many combined preparations with aspirin and paracetamol, but the dose used is often too small to contribute significantly to the analgesic potency of the preparation.

Dihydrocodeine

The derivative dihydrocodeine is quite widely used as a moderate analgesic. Side effects of dizziness, nausea, vomiting and gastro-intestinal disturbance, especially constipation, are sufficiently common to restrict its use to only a very few ambulant patients. The parenteral form, given by intramuscular injection, is occasionally used to control severe pain in patients in hospital.

Dihydrocodeine	
Advantages	Disadvantages
Effective analgesic May be given parenterally	Side effects preclude general use, especially in ambulant patients

Chart 5

Pentazocine

This is a relatively new analgesic which is claimed to be as effective as pethidine or morphine. It is occasionally used to supplement the analgesic/anti-inflammatory drugs in patients with severe pain especially those in hospital. Despite its claimed potency it does not produce addiction and is not, therefore, classified as a controlled drug. In general, however, it has proved disappointing in the treatment of pain of rheumatic origin. Side effects include drowsiness, which may prevent patients carrying on their normal jobs, hallucinations, nausea and vomiting.

```
                          Pentazocine
       Advantages                      Disadvantages
       Moderate analgesic              Disappointing in
       May be given parenterally         rheumatic patients
       Not subject to dangerous
         drugs legislation
```
Chart 6

Pethidine, morphine and other opiates

These have a very small place in the treatment of rheumatic diseases. Parenteral pethidine is occasionally used before or after painful splintage procedures and post-operatively. Because of the possibility of addiction, pethidine and other opiates are never given as routine drugs for the treatment of pain in rheumatic diseases.

```
                  Pethidine and other opiates
       Advantages                      Disadvantages
       Good analgesia                  ADDICTIVE—SHOULD
                                         NOT BE GENERALLY
                                         USED
```
Chart 7

Analgesic/Anti-inflammatory Drugs

As the name of this group of drugs implies, they combine pain relief with an anti-inflammatory action. They are the most widely used group of drugs in the rheumatic diseases.

Salicylates

Aspirin is the most widely used of the analgesic/anti-inflammatory preparations and is usually considered as the yardstick against which the effectiveness of other drugs is measured. Although aspirin is an analgesic at all doses, it is important to remember that it is only an anti-inflammatory drug in doses of 4 g per day or more. This is shown most dramatically in the treatment of rheumatic fever, where a high dose of aspirin—but not a low dose—causes a rapid decrease in temperature and ESR. In doses less than 4 g daily it is used entirely as an analgesic. The point is frequently not grasped by patients, who complain of their being given 'only aspirin' having previously taken inadequate doses.

Side effects. Unfortunately almost one-third of patients cannot tolerate aspirin. The main side effects are gastro-intestinal upset comprising indigestion, heartburn, nausea and vomiting. Aspirin must be used with caution in patients with a history of indigestion. It causes bleeding from the gastric mucosa and may precipitate severe haemorrhage in patients with peptic ulcers. About 70% of people taking aspirin will have a blood loss of 4-8 ml per day as a result of therapy. Many patients complain of being 'allergic' to aspirin. By this they usually mean that aspirin upsets their stomach. True aspirin hypersensitivity, which usually presents as giant urticaria, is extremely rare.

The other side effects of aspirin are those of overdosage—aspirin toxicity. Unfortunately, the anti-inflammatory dose of aspirin is very near the toxic dose, and patients with acute rheumatoid arthritis who are treated with high doses of aspirin may develop tinnitus (buzzing or ringing in the ears) or deafness, which resolves when the dose of aspirin is reduced. In children with rheumatic fever who may not be able to complain of the symptoms of overdosage, it is usual to measure the blood level of salicylate to control treatment. Aspirin also has a mild anti-coagulant effect and should not be used in patients with bleeding disorders such as haemophilia. It also reacts with anti-coagulants in the blood and so should never be given to patients on anti-coagulant therapy.

Aspirin

Advantages	*Disadvantages*
Effective analgesic	Frequent gastro-intestinal upset
Effective anti-inflammatory agent in doses of 4 g+ per day	Gastro-intestinal bleeding Mild anti-coagulant
Many preparations available to combat intolerance	
True hypersensitivity very rare	

The most commonly used and most useful anti-rheumatic preparation

Chart 8

Salicylate preparations. In order to reduce the incidence of side effects a large number of salicylate preparations are available. Gastric bleeding appears to be most common with plain aspirin tablets, and the use of *soluble aspirin* as the first preparation is almost universal. Each tablet contains 300 mg aspirin. If soluble aspirin causes gastro-intestinal upset several alternative preparations are available. *Enteric coated aspirin* is available as 325 mg and 650 mg tablets, the enteric coating being designed to resist digestion by gastric acid and release its contents in the more alkaline duodenum. *Glycine aspirin* is a combination of 600 mg aspirin with 300 mg glycine. This preparation dissolves in the mouth. It is doubtful if the amount of gastric bleeding caused by this preparation is any less than that with soluble aspirin, but the larger amount of aspirin in the tablet, its palatability and the fact that it can be taken without water continue to make it a useful preparation for patients at work. *Aloxiprin* is aluminium aspirin in 600 mg tablets. These may be swallowed, sucked or chewed, and may be dispersed in water. They may also be dispersed in milk, and many patients find this a very tolerable way of taking salicylates. There is some evidence that blood loss is less when taking aloxiprin than soluble aspirin. *Microencapsulated* aspirin is a relatively new preparation in which the aspirin is contained within tiny cellulose balls from which it diffuses when placed in liquids such as gastric and intestinal contents. The rate at which the aspirin diffuses out of the spheres is dependent on their thickness. By varying the size of the spheres it can be assured that all the aspirin is not released at one point, minimising local irritant action.

By using the various preparations of salicylate available, a satisfactory form can be found for most patients with rheumatic disease.

The dose of salicylate varies considerably depending on the nature and stage of the disease being treated. In conditions such as osteo-arthrosis or muscular rheumatism it is usually sufficient to tailor the dose to the patient's need for pain relief. In rheumatoid arthritis it is usual to aim at a dose of about 4 g per day in order to use the anti-inflammatory action of the drug. In acute rheumatoid arthritis and in acute rheumatism (rheumatic fever) it is usual to increase the dose until the patient suffers early symptoms of salicylate toxicity and then to reduce the dose slightly so that the patient is maintained on the highest possible dose below the toxic one. This ensures that maximum analgesic and anti-inflammatory effect is obtained.

Phenylbutazone

This is a member of the group of analgesic/anti-inflammatory drugs known as pyrazoles. The two most important are phenylbutazone and oxyphenbutazone. These are effective analgesic and anti-inflammatory drugs which are very widely used for both locomotor disorders and in the treatment of superficial thrombophlebitis. The effectiveness of the pyrazoles appears to be greater in ankylosing spondylitis than in other conditions. This effect is so striking that the administration of phenylbutazone is sometimes used as a therapeutic test when trying to diagnose early cases of ankylosing spondylitis.

Side effects are divided into two major categories—effects on the gastro-intestinal system and the bone marrow. Gastro-intestinal bleeding may be a major problem with pyrazoles, as may indigestion, heartburn and nausea. These problems may be partly overcome by the administration of the pyrazoles as suppositories, but the drugs are re-secreted into the stomach and may occasionally cause upper intestinal symptoms even when administered rectally. Buffered and enteric coated tablets decrease the incidence of dyspepsia, but have not abolished it. The effects on the bone marrow are two-fold. An agranulocytosis may develop, in which there is failure of formation of the granulocytes (neutrophil leucocytes, eosinophils and basophils) in the bone marrow. This leaves the patient without defence against infection and is almost invariably fatal. This condition may occur after only a short course of treatment. It appears to be hypersensitive ('allergic') in nature, and may affect young patients. The second effect on the bone marrow is the production of a hypoplastic anaemia. In this condition the drug appears to 'poison' the marrow causing a generalised diminution in cell formation. This affects all cell types, both red and white, and platelets. If untreated it may continue to a total aplasia, in which cell formation by the marrow ceases altogether. This complication occurs in elderly patients (aged 55 or more) and appears to be dose-dependent, that is the larger the dose taken the more the chance of its occurring. Treatment is by the withdrawal of the drug immediately blood counts show the condition is starting, supplemented by blood transfusion and anabolic steroids or corticosteroids as necessary. This condition too may be lethal. It must be emphasised, however, that both these complications are rare, although they limit the usefulness of an effective group of drugs.

Phenylbutazone and oxyphenbutazone

Advantages	Disadvantages
Effective analgesics	Gastro-intestinal bleeding
Effective anti-inflammatory agents	Agranulocytosis
Enhanced effect in ankylosing spondylitis	Aplastic anaemia

Chart 9

Lesser side effects include a tendency to cause fluid retention, which means that care has to be taken in giving these drugs to patients with cardiac failure or renal disease. Skin rashes may also occur. There is no difference between phenylbutazone and oxyphenbutazone in the incidence of side effects.

Preparations include 100 mg and 200 mg tablets of phenylbutazone and 100 mg tablets of oxyphenbutazone. It is usually considered inadvisable to give a dose of more than 600 mg daily of the tablets. Suppositories containing 250 mg of each preparation are available. Phenylbutazone injection (600 mg) is extremely painful and is, therefore, compounded with the local anaesthetic xylocaine.

Indomethacin

Indomethacin is a widely used analgesic/anti-inflammatory agent. Its potency is equivalent to that of phenylbutazone and it is used in similar clinical situations. It is often advised to give it with milk.

Side effects include gastro-intestinal upset and bleeding and severe pounding headaches. Other side effects such as rashes occur less commonly. Indomethacin is made in 25 mg and 50 mg capsules and 100 mg suppositories. The suppositories are particularly useful in the treatment of morning stiffness, being inserted at night and maintaining their effect in the morning. The same dose given by mouth is as effective if it can be tolerated. Very high doses are used in the treatment of acute gout. Indomethacin is probably the most widely used analgesic/anti-inflammatory drug after aspirin. Doses range from 50 mg to 250 mg daily.

	Indomethacin
Advantages	*Disadvantages*
Effective analgesic and anti-inflammatory agent	Headaches
	Gastro-intestinal upset
Available as capsules or suppositories	

Chart 10

Fenamates

The fenamates, mefanamic acid and flufenamic acid, are effective analgesic/anti-inflammatory agents. *Side effects* include a high incidence of gastro-intestinal upset, especially diarrhoea.

Benorylate

This is a recently introduced preparation which is a chemical combination of aspirin and paracetamol. The benorylate does not break down into its two constituents until it reaches the bloodstream, and thus gives aspirin therapy with no direct gastric irritation. Its prolonged action means that it need be given only twice daily, and its liquid form is highly acceptable to some patients. Gastro-intestinal upset does occur, and symptoms of salicylate overdosage, such as tinnitus and deafness, occur not infrequently as the usual dose (10 ml b.d.) is equivalent to 4 g of aspirin. A tablet form has been recently introduced.

Propionic acid derivatives

This series of drugs is the most recently introduced in the treatment of rheumatic diseases. The first was *Ibuprofen* which is a mild analgesic with some anti-inflammatory effect. Gastro-intestinal upset and bleeding is uncommon in doses up to 800 mg daily, but these doses are relatively ineffective in rheumatic diseases. Higher doses increase the efficacy a little but also increase the side effects.

Fenoprofen was originally marketed as capsules, but these have now been replaced by tablets which are easier to swallow. It is similar to Ibuprofen in its tolerance, but appears to be a little more effective. The dose is one to two 300 mg tablets 3-4 times daily.

Ketoprofen is similar to fenoprofen, but is supplied in 50 mg capsules, the dose again being up to two four times daily.

Naproxen appears to be the most potent of the propionic acid derivatives and has the advantage of twice daily administration. The standard dose is one 250 mg tablet twice daily, though up to two tablets twice daily may be needed, especially in the treatment of osteoarthrosis.

Azapropazone

This is a recently introduced agent which in doses of 900-1200 mg daily appears to combine reasonable efficacy with a low incidence of side effects.

Anti-inflammatory Drugs

This group of drugs has no direct analgesic effect. Their action is entirely limited to reducing the inflammation taking place in joints or other tissues. It follows, therefore, that they have no place in the treatment of non-inflammatory diseases such as osteoarthrosis.

Corticosteroids

The corticosteroids are the most powerful members of the anti-inflammatory group. They are all based on the natural hormones, principally cortisone and hydrocortisone, made by cells in the adrenal cortex. There are two ways of giving increased amounts of corticosteroids. Either the patient's own adrenals may be stimulated to overproduce the natural hormones, or synthetic substitutes may be given by mouth or injection.

The normal adrenal gland has the amount of hormone released from it controlled through a series of 'feedback' mechanisms, the other component being the adrenocorticotrophic hormone of the anterior pituitary gland. If ACTH is injected into a patient the adrenals will produce excessive amounts of cortisone and hydrocortisone, which will have an anti-inflammatory effect. Apart from producing the other side effects of steroid therapy (discussed below) this method of treatment has the additional disadvantage of requiring injections. The 'pituitary-adrenal axis' is better maintained by ACTH treatment than by oral corticosteroids. Patients with conditions such as asthma may give their own ACTH injections subcutaneously, but the sort of patients with rheumatoid arthritis sufficiently severe to need corticosteroid therapy are rarely able to cope with self-injection.

ACTH	
Advantages	*Disadvantages*
Powerful anti-inflammatory effect	Drawbacks of steroid therapy *plus* increased pigmentation; need for injections and reactions to foreign protein

Chart 11

The interval between injections may be reduced by using a depot preparation from which the ACTH is released slowly. Recently the active part of the ACTH molecule (tetracosactrin) has been manufactured instead of the entire hormone being extracted from animals. This makes dosage more precise and reduces the likelihood of hypersensitivity reactions caused by injecting animal protein. In practice reactions appear to be almost as common, and some patients develop marked pigmentation of the skin. One occasional use for ACTH is to give it to the patient in an intravenous infusion. This may help the patient to get over a severe exacerbation more quickly, and may also be used to assess their response to future oral corticosteroid therapy. A good response to intravenous ACTH suggests that a good response may be expected if oral corticosteroids are given.

The use of synthetic corticosteroids is more widespread than the use of ACTH. These drugs are more powerful in their anti-inflammatory effects and offer the convenience of oral dosage.

Side effects of corticosteroids
1. Suppression of response to stress
2. Osteoporosis
3. Thinning of skin
4. Moon face
5. Buffalo hump
6. Redistribution of body-fat—thin limbs and fat trunk
7. Striae
8. Fluid retention
9. Hypertension
10. Altered glucose tolerance; diabetes mellitus
11. Increased liability to infections
12. Cataract formation
13. Muscle weakness and myopathy
14. Intestinal ulceration
15. Psychosis

Chart 12

Side effects of corticosteroids are numerous, and some are listed in Chart 12. The suppression of the response to stress is due to the fact that the normal adrenal produces more cortisone and hydrocortisone in response to injury or other stress. The administration of oral corticosteroids causes atrophy of the adrenal cortex with the result that the normal response to stress is lost. For this reason all patients taking corticosteroids should carry a card giving details of the drug they are taking. It is most important that patients taking corticosteroids are given these cards. If they are subjected to any extra stress, such as an accident or operation, they are given intravenous hydrocortisone to compensate for the loss of a normal stress response when they would produce more cortisone and hydrocortisone for themselves.

Corticosteroid preparations. There are many synthetic corticosteroid preparations and new ones appear each year. The object of the newer drugs is to increase the amount of anti-inflammatory activity while decreasing the other, unwanted, effects. In general this is not successful and prednisone and prednisolone remain the most frequently used preparations. The standard tablets are 5 mg, but 1 mg tablets are available, which are useful in making small changes in the dose. In patients with gastric intolerance, enteric coated prednisolone is given in 2.5 mg tablets. If the patient is unable to take tablets, such as following gastric surgery or during the treatment of severe haematemesis, prednisolone may be given by intramuscular injection.

The dose used is the smallest possible which relieves the patient's symptoms. In general 10 mg per day or less of prednisolone is given, as side effects appear to be decreased by using this dose.

In children with Still's disease the use of corticosteroids has been associated with stunting of growth. This problem has been lessened by the use of alternate day corticosteroid therapy. The total dose remains the same, but the stunting effect of, for example, 10 mg prednisolone on alternate days is less than that of 5 mg daily.

Intra-articular corticosteroids. Corticosteroids may be injected directly into the joint in an attempt to increase the concentration at the inflamed synovium. This is the same principle as applying corticosteroid creams to inflamed skin. Intra-articular injections must be given using an aseptic technique, as accidental infection of the joint may be catastrophic. It is also important that the intra-articular preparation of the injected corticosteroid is used. If intravenous hydrocortisone is put into joints, absorption from the joint is so rapid that it is ineffective, and any crystals retained in the joint may cause an acute synovitis similar to acute gout. When weightbearing joints are injected, the patient must rest for forty eight hours after injection. This prevents over-use of the joint which may cause great damage to it. Similar damage, called steroid arthropathy, may also occur in any joint into which corticosteroid injections are made too frequently.

The usual intra-articular preparation is of hydrocortisone acetate, 25 mg in 1 ml. The dose depends on the size of the joint, varying from 5 mg into inter-phalangeal joints to 50 mg into knees. Other intra-articular corticosteroid preparations have, in general, no advantages over hydrocortisone, except that the smaller volume needed may be advantageous in injecting small joints. Recently the problems of introducing needles into small joints have been removed by the use of needle-less injectors, such as those used for mass vaccination.

Gold

Gold is widely used as an anti-inflammatory drug in the treatment of rheumatoid arthritis. It is given by intra-muscular injection, at weekly intervals initially. The first two injections are small, being test doses.

Drug Therapy in Rheumatic Diseases 217

Thereafter the traditional 'course' of gold was to give 50 mg weekly until a total of 1 g had been given, then to stop. It was found that second courses of gold, given after an interval, were rarely as effective as the first course. Two dosage schedules have been used to overcome this disadvantage. The gold may be given in 50 mg doses weekly until 1 g is reached, then fortnightly for two months, three-weekly for three months, monthly for four months and four to six weekly thereafter. Alternatively a weekly dose of 20 mg is given, which may be reduced to fortnightly once the full effect has occurred, but is thereafter continued indefinitely. There is usually a latent period of about three months after the first injection before the effect of gold becomes apparent.

Side effects of gold may be severe, and occur in about one third of patients. The main ones are effects on the skin, the bone marrow, usually agranulocytosis, and the kidney. If the blood count becomes abnormal, or the patient develops an irritable skin rash or albuminuria the gold should be stopped. It is important to ask the patient on each occasion a gold injection is given whether they have developed a rash.

A urine specimen must be tested and be free of albumin before each injection is given.

Gold

Advantages	*Disadvantages*
Effective long-term anti-inflammatory agent	Toxic effects involving marrow, skin, or kidney in one third of patients. Need for injection
ALWAYS CHECK THE URINE BEFORE GIVING GOLD INJECTIONS	

Chart 13

Only one preparation of gold, sodium aurothiomalate ('Myocrisin') is available, in ampoules containing 1 mg, 5 mg, 10 mg, 20 mg and 50 mg.

Antimalarial drugs

Antimalarial drugs, chloroquine and hydroxychloroquine, are occasionally used in the treatment of rheumatoid arthritis. They have a mild anti-inflammatory effect, but their use is limited by the development of retinal damage which may cause irreversible blindness. For this reason patients should have regular eye examinations when on long-term treatment.

	Antimalarials	
Advantages		*Disadvantages*
Mild anti-inflammatory agent		Potentially severe ocular toxicity reduces use

Chart 14

Muscle Relaxants

Muscle spasm is often present in patients with rheumatic disorders, and relief of spasm is usually achieved by pain relief. Combined preparations are available which contain muscle relaxants, but these are rarely useful. *Diazepam* is used in some conditions with muscle spasm, especially those in which there is an element of anxiety as well, as it is a mild tranquilliser. Given intravenously, diazepam is valuable in reducing muscle spasm around a joint when splints are being applied. In this way a knee may be made much straighter before serial plasters are applied by reducing the spasm in surrounding muscles. *Methocarbamol* is sometimes used either alone or combined with aspirin in the treatment of back pain.

Psychiatric Drugs

Prolonged painful and disabling diseases produce anxiety and depression in the patients who suffer from them. Treatment both with minor tranquillisers and anti-depressant drugs may be needed as a part of the patient's treatment. Physical complaints may be the 'respectable' way for a patient to bring psychiatric problems to the attention of the doctor, in which case treatment of the primary psychiatric disorder is indicated.

Haematinics

Anaemia in rheumatoid arthritis sometimes needs treatment with iron. This frequently has to be given by injection, either intramuscular or intravenous. Both methods of injection require special precautions. Intramuscular iron must be given using the Z-track injection technique otherwise staining of the skin occurs due to the iron leaking back along the needle track (Fig. 21.1). Apart from being unsightly, this has been held to be negligent, as necrosis can occur. Intravenous iron may be given by total dose infusion, in which the whole amount of iron needed to correct the anaemia and replace iron stores in the body is given in an intravenous infusion, or by direct intravenous injections, on alternate days over a period of two to three weeks. During and after both types of injection the patients must be carefully observed as rarely an acute collapse may take place due to hypersensitivity to the injection. Following total dose infusions patients should rest for at least twenty four hours. If they are allowed up immediately an acute flare-up of the joint may occur, although some patients feel that their joints are improved by this procedure.

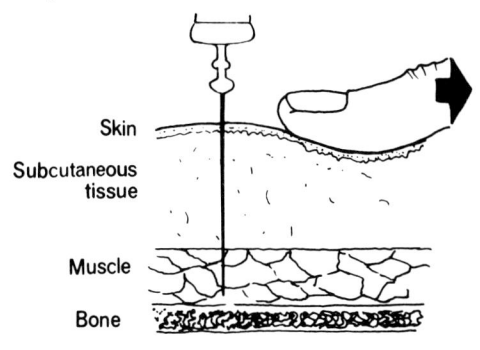

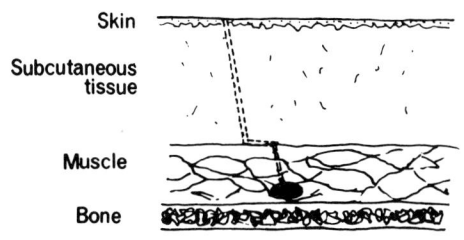

Fig. 21.1. Intra-muscular iron injection— Z track technique to prevent staining of skin.

New Forms of Therapy

Constant attempts are being made not only to improve the efficacy of currently available types of drugs but also to introduce new methods of treatment.

D-penicillamine

This has recently been found to be helpful in the treatment of rheumatoid arthritis. It appears to retard the progress of the disease producing a fall in ESR and reduction in titre of the SCAT. Side effects are common and include albuminuria, rashes, gastro-intestinal upset, loss of taste and blood dyscrasias, especially thrombocytopaenia. For this reason careful supervision has to be undertaken and frequent blood tests are needed. The patients must be warned that little or no effect of penicillamine treatment will become apparent for at least three months, and that maximum benefit will not be apparent for about a year. With currently used dose schedules approximately 50% of patients have to withdraw from this therapy because of side effects, but it has been suggested that lower doses and more cautious introduction of therapy may allow more patients to continue on treatment. Because of the risks involved, penicillamine therapy has to be strictly controlled.

Immunosuppressive drugs

This also applies to the immunosuppressive drugs which have been used in patients with severe rheumatoid arthritis. They have been found to decrease the amount of corticosteroid which the patient needs to take, and may cause some improvement by their own action. The reason for introducing these drugs was the suggestion that rheumatoid arthritis was a disorder of the immune system of the body. The immunosuppressive drugs do not, however, appear to act by their effect on the immune system.

Glossary of Drugs

This list is not exhaustive, but lists the main examples of each type of analgesic and anti-inflammatory drug, mentioned in their order in which they appear in the text.

Analgesics

    Paracetamol — Panadol, Calpol, PCM, Tabalgin, Ticelgesic

    Phenacetin. PREPARATIONS CONTAINING PHENACETIN SHOULD NOT BE USED. THESE INCLUDE: Sonalgin, Dexocodene, Saridone, Orgraine

Dextropropoxyphene	Doloxene Depronal
Dextropropoxyphene and paracetamol	Distalgesic

Codeine tablets are rarely used alone in the treatment of pain, being reserved for the symptomatic treatment of diarrhoea. Combinations with other mild analgesics include:

with aspirin	Codis Analgin Antoin
with paracetamol	Solpadeine Panadeine Co Medocodene Paracodol Parake Paralgin Para-seltzer
Dihydrocodeine	DF 118
Pentazocine	Fortral

Analgesic/Anti-inflammatory Agents

Aspirin	Tasprin
Soluble aspirin	Solprin Bufferin Claradin
Enteric coated aspirin	Nu-seals aspirin Safapryn (in paracetamol coating)
Glycine aspirin	Paynocil
Aloxiprin	Palaprin Forte
Micro-encapsulated aspirin	Levius

Phenylbutazone	Butazolidin
	Butaphen
	Butazone
	Ethibute
	Flexazone
— *enteric coated*	Butacote
— *buffered*	Butazolidin Alka
Oxyphenbutazone	Tanderil
— *enteric coated*	Tandacote
— *buffered*	Tanderil Alka
Indomethacin	Indocid
	Imbrilon
Mefenamic acid	Ponstan
Flufenamic acid	Arlef
Benorylate	Benoral
Ibuprofen	Brufen
Fenoprofen	Fenopron
Ketoprofen	Orudis
Naproxen	Naprosyn
Alclofenac	Prinalgin
Azapropazone	Rheumox

22
Surgery

Definitions
Soft Tissue Procedures
Operations on Joints
  Arthrotomy
  Debridement
  Synovectomy
  Osteotomy
  Excision arthroplasty
  Hemiarthroplasty
  Total arthroplasty
  Arthrodesis
Factors affecting Surgery
  Pain
  Disability
  Age
  Stage of the disease
  Joint involved
  Overall mobility
  Extent of disease
  Home circumstances
  Other medical conditions
  Demands of work
  Treatment with corticosteroids
  Personality
Complications
Nursing Aspects

The biggest advances in the treatment of arthritic conditions over the past two decades have been in the realm of surgery. This is particularly true in the development of an adequate total replacement for the hip joint. This has alleviated the suffering of thousands of patients with osteoarthrosis of that joint. Another major advance has been in the setting up throughout the United Kingdom of Combined Rheumatic-

Orthopaedic clinics, in which rheumatologists and orthopaedic surgeons discuss the management of rheumatic patients with particular reference to surgery. The pre-operative and post-operative management of these patients, particularly where major surgery is undertaken, is as important as the surgery itself and should also be jointly supervised.

Definitions

A number of definitions are helpful in understanding this subject.

Arthrodesis — the surgical fixation of a joint by fusion of the joint surfaces. It is an artificially created ankylosis.

Arthroplasty — operation on a joint to form a new joint. Sometimes this is by cutting off the end(s) of the adjacent bones and allowing fibrous tissue to grow between the surfaces (excision arthroplasty). Sometimes it is by replacing one worn joint surface with metal or plastic (hemi-arthroplasty), and sometimes by replacing both joint surfaces (total arthroplasty).

Arthrotomy — surgical incision of a joint.

Debridement — the removal of foreign matter and devitalised tissue.

-ectomy — the removal of whatever precedes the ending. For example, a patellectomy is the removal of the patella.

Osteotomy — the surgical cutting of a bone (in this context it is usually right across the bone).

Synovectomy — the removal of synovium from around the joint. It is never possible to remove this completely.

Tenotomy — the division of a tendon.

Soft Tissue Procedures

Decompression operations may bring great relief to the patient. The most commonly performed is median nerve decompression for a carpal tunnel syndrome. The median nerve is compressed in the carpal tunnel on the palmar aspect of the wrist. The patient often has disabling symptoms which are worse at night and consist of severe pins and needles and numbness of the thumb, index, middle and half the ring finger. Sometimes there is pain up the arm. The condition is completely

Surgery

relieved by division of the carpal ligament over the carpal tunnel. The operation is usually done as a day case. It can, if necessary, be done under local anaesthetic, should the patient's general condition not warrant a general anaesthetic. The scar is barely visible after a few months. Sometimes the ulnar nerve is trapped at the elbow or compressed. An ulnar nerve decompression has similar gratifying results. There is a much less common condition in the foot comparable to the carpal tunnel syndrome, called the tarsal tunnel syndrome, and this likewise responds to simple surgery.

Subcutaneous nodules may be troublesome or unsightly and are sometimes removed. They have a tendency to recur, however.

Cysts are sometimes excised. A Baker's cyst protruding from the posterior aspect of the synovial membrane of the knee in the popliteal fossa may cause compression of structures such as veins, and may track down into the calf, where it may rupture. Attempts should be made to aspirate this first and inject local hydrocortisone. If the cyst recurs after this procedure has been adopted on two or three occasions, excision may be required. Some surgeons advocate an anterior synovectomy for the treatment of this, however, since in rheumatoid patients the cyst communicates with the knee joint by a valve-like mechanism.

Occasionally tendons are severed where they appear to be causing a contraction of the joint (e.g. the hip or knee). Such operations rarely produce much relief of pain. Tendons may rupture and require repair. This occurs in the hand, particularly with the extensor muscles. If this is due to tenosynovitis which has invaded the tendon, then it is worth trying to achieve union by a Rancho splint (Fig. 22.1). The tendons join up with each other on the back of the wrist and hand, so that wearing the splint consistently for three months may cause them to unite

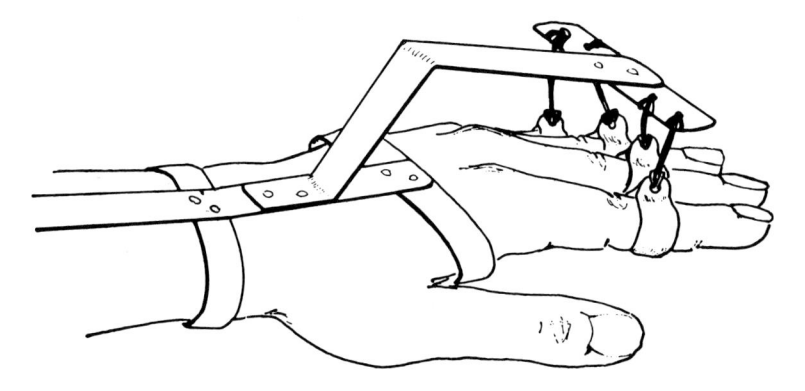

Fig. 22.1. Rancho splint.

spontaneously. If, however, this fails, or if the rupture is due to a rough ulnar styloid process which has abraded the tendon, then surgical repair and sometimes transplantation of a tendon to achieve the same function may be undertaken.

Operations on Joints

Table 22.1 shows the types of operations which are sometimes performed on various joints of the body.

Joint	Operations
Hip	Tenotomy, Arthrodesis, Osteotomy, Excision femoral head, Cup arthroplasty, Replacement femoral head, Total joint replacement.
Knee	Debridement, Synovectomy, Osteotomy, Patellectomy, Total joint replacement (hinge or mould), Arthrodesis.
Ankle	Synovectomy, Arthrodesis, Total replacement.
Metatarso-phalangeal joints	Bunionectomy, Keller's operation on 1st mtp, Fowler's operation on all mtps.
Toes	Proximal phalangectomy, Amputation.
Cervical Spine	Laminectomy, Fusion.
Shoulder	Synovectomy, Excision of acromial end, Excision of humeral head, Arthrodesis, Replacement humeral head, Total replacement.
Elbow	Synovectomy, Excision radial head, Hinge replacement.
Wrist	Excision lower end of ulna, Fusion.
Metacarpo-phalangeal joints	Synovectomy, Excision metacarpal heads, Hinge replacement of joint.
Proximal inter-phalangeal joint	Arthrodesis (especially of thumb). Hinge replacement.

Table 22.1 Operations which may be performed on various arthritic joints.

Arthrotomy

This is usually done to obtain a biopsy for diagnostic purposes. It is also used to insert an arthroscope so that the inside of the joint can be inspected directly. Sometimes the joint is washed out with saline (joint lavage) and occasional benefit ensues. This is particularly so if there is a lot of fibrin in the joint fluid and loosely attached to the synovial membrane.

Debridement

This is occasionally done in a knee where the x-rays suggest that there are loose fragments of cartilage or bone.

Synovectomy

This is most frequently done in the knee. It is undertaken for local arrest of the disease, for relief of pain, to remove mechanical obstructions, and occasionally for cosmetic reasons. About two-thirds of the patients get benefit from this procedure. It is best done before there are any erosions of the joint surface. If patients have gained and retained benefit for two years, they are likely to continue with this improvement. However, the synovium does regrow quickly after the operation and may be subject to involvement in a generalised flare up of the disease process.

Osteotomy

This used to be done frequently in the hip, but is more often reserved these days for the knee. In an extensive study which Dr J. M. Iveson and Mr E. B. Longton have done at Leeds, they have found that some 60% of the patients with osteoarthrosis and rheumatoid arthritis of the knees benefit from this procedure. A comparison has been made of single and double osteotomies. The single osteotomy employs a cut across the upper part of the tibia. The double osteotomy also has a cut across the lower end of the femur. The tibial osteotomy patients have done rather better, and those in whom there was a varus deformity (bow legs) have done particularly well. On the whole the patients with osteoarthrosis fared better than those with rheumatoid arthritis. When osteotomy is done at the hip this is often combined with fixing the bone in a new position (Fig. 22.2).

Excision arthroplasty

This may be done in joints such as the metacarpo-phalangeal joints (Vainio arthroplasty), the metatarso-phalangeal joints (Fowler's arthroplasty) (Fig. 22.3) and the elbow. We have analysed 414 cases of excision arthroplasty of the elbow in the literature and found 40% gave a good result, 30% a fair result, and 30% were failures. It is usually done for rheumatoid arthritis.

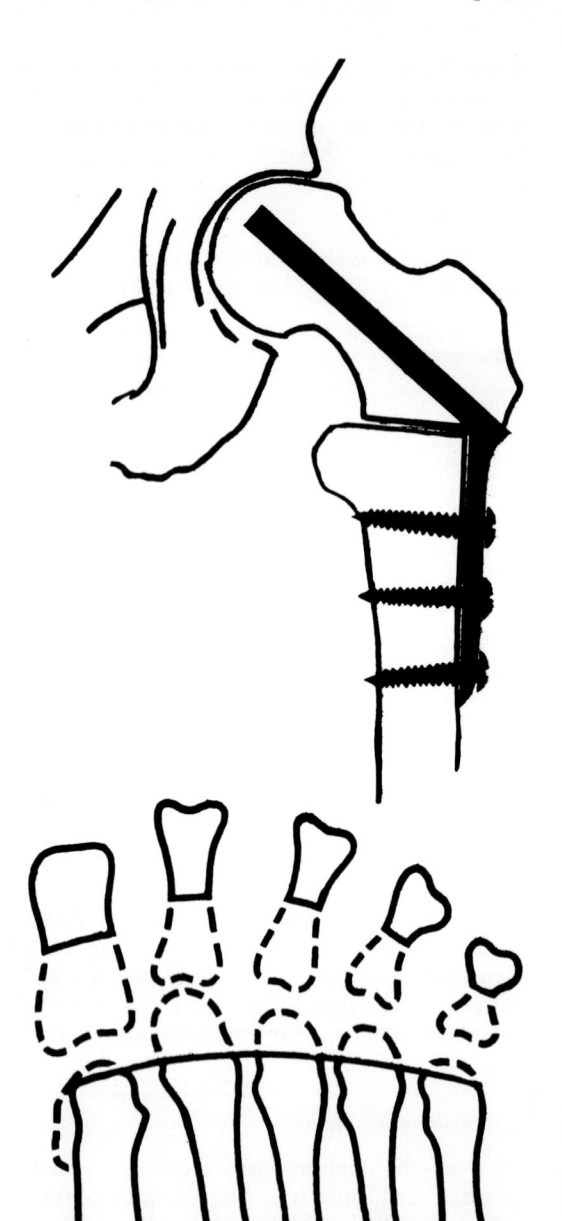

Fig. 22.2. McMurray osteotomy of hip.

Fig. 22.3. Fowler's arthroplasty of the forefoot.

Hemiarthroplasty

An example of this is the Austin Moore prosthesis, in which the femoral head is replaced by a metal prosthesis. Another example is the Mackintosh arthroplasty, which replaces one or both tibial plateaux with a metal disc.

Total arthroplasty

This has been developed to its highest degree in the hip, where it has revolutionised the lives of many patients. Two main types of arthroplasty are available. Firstly, the type in which the acetabulum is replaced by a metal cup and the head of the femur by a metal prosthesis. This is the basis of the McKee-Farrar arthroplasty (Fig. 22.4) and the Ring prosthesis. One of the main differences between the two is that the McKee-Farrar prosthesis is fixed in position with polymethylmethacrylate cement. The most widely used prosthesis today, however, is that in

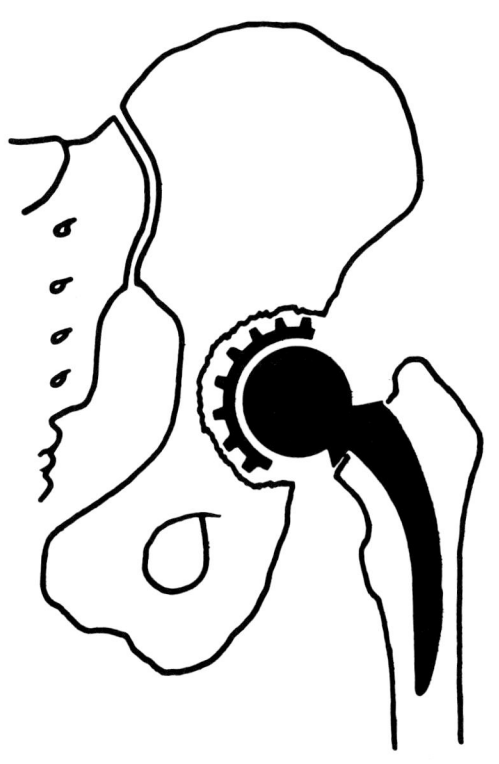

Fig. 22.4. McKee Farrar arthroplasty of the hip.

which a stainless steel femoral component articulates with a plastic hip socket of high density polyethylene. This has been developed by Professor Sir John Charnley at Wrightington Hospital, near Wigan.

Hinge arthroplasties have been used at the elbow and the knee, but on the whole are undesirable because they produce complications. They do not simulate closely the natural geometry or movement of the joint. They tend to loosen and to wear. Other types of knee replacement have used a metal mould at the lower end of the femur and a plastic replacement for the top of the tibia. This takes away much less bone and is better functionally. The prosthesis of this type developed at Leeds by Dr B. B. Seedhom and Mr E. B. Longton is shown in Fig. 22.5. The shoulder arthroplasty, developed in our Group by Mr B. Jobbins and Mr B. Reeves, is shown diagrammatically in Fig. 22.6.

Arthrodesis

In deciding between an arthrodesis and an arthroplasty consideration has to be given to the functional demands on the joint. This involves taking into consideration the joint affected, the extent of the disease, the overall mobility, and the age of the patient. In symmetrical arthritis, e.g. when both knees are affected, it is usually undesirable to arthrodese one, since extra strain will be put on the knee of the opposite leg, with deterioration. Prior to the development of knee arthroplasty, however, this was often the only possibility for very damaged joints.

Factors affecting Surgery

In considering the possibility of surgery and the type to be undertaken, many factors have to be considered.

Pain

The pain that the patient is experiencing is one major factor. When pain is present at night and wakens the patient, then surgery must be seriously considered, particularly if it has not responded to a full regime of conservative therapy including treatment in hospital.

Disability

The disability of the patient must also be considered. Severe involvement of the hip may make toilet functions extremely difficult and sexual activity impossible. This may be a good reason for replacement arthroplasty.

Surgery

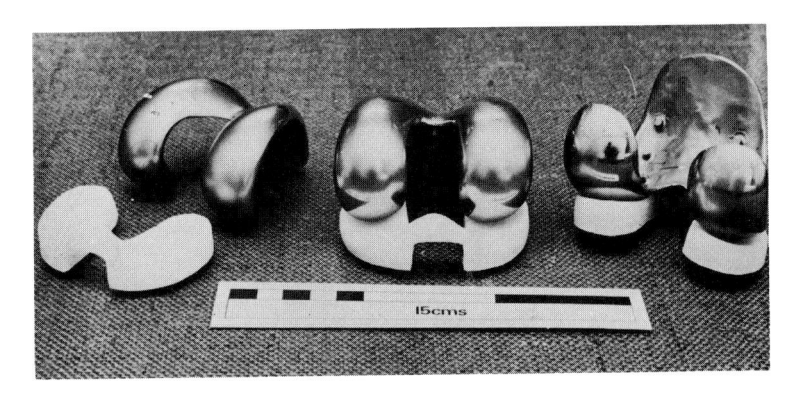

Fig. 22.5. Leeds knee arthroplasty.

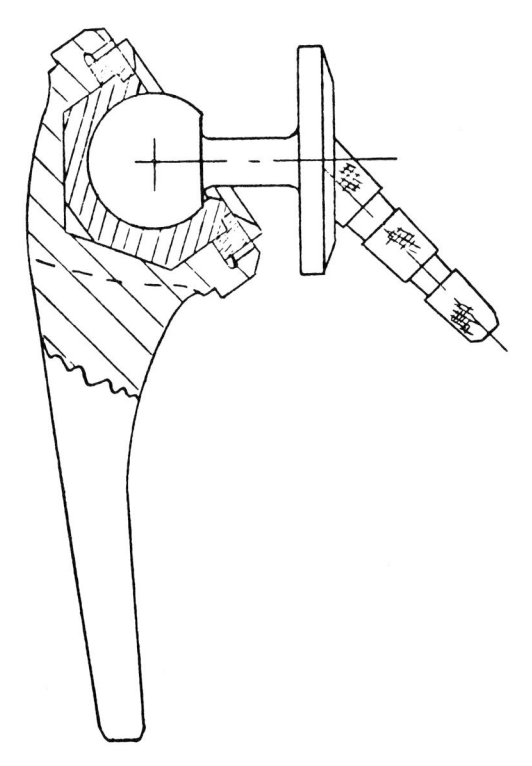

Fig. 22.6. Leeds shoulder prosthesis.

Age

The age of the patient may induce caution in replacement arthroplasties, which have only been evaluated over a period of fifteen years. Surgeons are often reluctant therefore, to put such joints in younger people. In general age is no bar to surgery.

Stage of the disease

The stage of the disease will have a direct bearing on the type of operation advocated. In early rheumatoid disease synovectomy is usually the treatment of choice.

Joint involved

The joint involved will also dictate the type of surgery. Subluxated metatarso-phalangeal joints which are giving a good deal of pain, not relieved by appropriate footwear, are usually best treated by excision of the metatarsal heads. At the wrist, however, fusion is the operation of choice. Here good function can be achieved even though the wrist is fixed.

Overall mobility

The overall mobility will be a factor in the situation. The patient who is confined to a wheel chair, but is experiencing considerable pain in the hips, will be grateful for an excision arthroplasty of the hips, in which the femoral heads are removed (Girdlestone arthroplasty). Stability will have been lost, but pain will have been relieved.

Extent of the disease

The extent of the disease may limit the amount of surgery. A single joint operation may not benefit the patient with widespread involvement of other weightbearing joints by rheumatoid disease.

Home circumstances

Home circumstances are important. The woman living on her own with bilateral median nerve compression should only have one operation at a time, if surgery is being undertaken as a day case. Inadequate home circumstances may also require the mobilisation of community services to help the patient during the period of convalescence and rehabilitation.

Other medical conditions

These will modify the approach to surgery. Severe disease elsewhere may necessitate surgery such as carpal tunnel decompression being done under local anaesthetic. Cardiac failure may limit the exercise tolerance of the patient, so that increasing mobility is no longer a factor to be considered in the possibility of joint surgery—quite apart from the risk of a major operation.

Demands of work

The demands of work will influence surgery in that much standing and loading of weightbearing joints causes hesitation in the use of total joint arthroplasty, particularly in younger patients.

Treatment with corticosteroids

This must be carefully noted. Because of the danger of collapse during or after the operation from adrenal insufficiency, such patients are operated on in hospital. Additional steroids are given before, during and after surgery. Intramuscular or intravenous steroids should be available for administration should collapse occur. These are rarely needed however, and previous corticosteroid therapy is not a contra-indication to surgery.

Personality

The personality of the sufferer will have a profound effect on the rehabilitation after surgery. It is rarely advisable to persuade a timid, diffident patient to submit to surgery. The ones who do best are those with plenty of 'go'.

Complications

The major hazard of surgery is infection. If this is deep-seated it usually requires the removal of a prosthesis. Deep vein thrombosis and pulmonary embolus are particular hazards in lower limb surgery and may be fatal. Wound healing tends to be delayed in patients with rheumatoid arthritis. This is mainly due to haematoma formation. The problems of healing do not seem to be related to treatment with steroids.

When osteotomy is performed failure of the bone to unite may be a rare complication. There may also be loss of movement post-operatively and persistent encouragement and physiotherapy may be required to regain the mobility of a knee. Sometimes there is a flexion deformity, or an inability fully to extend the leg actively, although it can be done passively (extension lag). This often persists if it has been present prior to operation. For this reason pre-operative physiotherapy is important. If bones are realigned, e.g. the correction of a varus deformity of the knee (knock-knees), pressure on adjacent nerves may result. In the knee this can produce a common peroneal (lateral popliteal) nerve palsy.

Nursing Aspects

It is important that pre-operatively the patient should be fully assessed physically, psychologically and functionally. The functional assessment may well be made by the occupational therapist as far as the activities of daily living are concerned. This will help to assess the benefit of the operation, and also to ascertain any particular problems that may arise due to other joint difficulties. Certain deformities may be overcome before operation—for example a flexion deformity of the knee. The muscles should be strengthened where possible, particularly the quadriceps muscle. The operation should be explained to the patients and particularly the length of time they are likely to be in hospital, and the length of time that they will have added difficulties at home, due to being either in plaster or bandages.

Post-operatively, on return from the theatre, the limb should be elevated and positioned properly. The bandages will require to be checked and a record will be kept of the temperature, pulse and respiration, with a note of the blood pressure. The limb will be checked for bleeding and any intravenous infusion and drainage tubes also checked. From this point onwards, careful watch will be kept for development of chest infection or deep vein thrombosis in the leg. Chest physiotherapy will be given and the nurse will assist in this as well as in the exercises of the limbs at the appropriate time, particularly the quadriceps muscles. Watch should be kept for any circulatory changes, especially if a plaster has been applied, and any pressure sores avoided. Post-operational blood tests and x-rays will be done. The time of mobilisation of the joint will depend on the nature of the procedure and the policy of the surgeon. There is a tendency to earlier mobilisation post-operatively. It may be necessary to re-order shoes made-to-measure after operations on the feet and after operations which realign the legs. For a more detailed account of orthopaedic nursing, standard works such as *Orthopaedics for Nurses* by A. Naylor should be consulted.

Index

Achilles tendinitis, 129, 133
Acromio-clavicular joint, 93
ACTH, 200, 201, 214, 215
Acute rheumatism, 107
Age factor, 168, 232
Agglutination tests, 22, 30, 187
Albumin, 200, 217
   test for, 188
Albuminuria, 188, 199, 201
Alcohol, 177, 196
Alkaline phosphatase, 187
Allopurinol, 124, 177
Aloxiprin, 210
Amyloidosis, 28, 199
Anaemia, 31, 44, 61, 218
Analgesics, 205-8, 220
Ankle
   joint mobilisation, 157
   twisted, 82
Ankle disease, 127
Ankylosing spondylitis, 13, 14, 29, 56-64, 89, 129, 132, 135, 138, 139, 155, 168, 174, 178, 182
   age of onset, 57
   blood tests, 61
   clinical features, 57
   complications, 61
   occupational therapy, 162
   pain radiation, 59
   pathology, 56
   physical signs, 59
   physiotherapy, 144-45
   presenting features, 58
   prevalence, 57
   prognosis, 61
   spinal changes, 61
   stoop, 59
   treatment, 63-64
   variant of, 48
   X-ray changes, 61
Antibiotics, 55
Antimalarial drugs, 99, 138, 217

Antinuclear factor, 102, 104
Anti-streptolysin O (ASO), 111, 188
Anxiety, 95, 169, 199, 218
Arthralgia, 47, 98
Arthritis, 13, 19, 48
   migratory, 109
   miscellaneous types, 135-43
Arthritis and Rheumatism Council, 44, 64, 125, 174
Arthrodesis, 224, 230
Arthroplasty, 45, 131, 224, 227
Arthroscopy, 193, 201
Arthrotomy, 224, 226
Aschoff's nodes, 109
Aspiration, 53, 55, 189, 200
Aspirin, 123, 206, 208-10, 218
Austin Moore prosthesis, 229
Auto-immunity, 23
Azapropazone, 213

Back pain, 18, 65, 69, 78, 80, 87, 151, 218
Baclofen, 80
Baker's cyst, 225
Ball and socket (spheroidal) joint, 4
'Bamboo spine', 63
Barium studies, 192
Bathing and bathing aids, 157, 164, 165, 175
Beat knee, 18, 85
Benorylate, 213
β haemolytic streptococci, 107
Bicipital tendinitis, 92
Bicipital tendon, 9
Blood culture, 188
Blood supply, 7
Blood tests, 30, 99, 184, 220
Boosted lubrication, 11
Bornholm disease, 48, 87
Bouchard's nodes, 39
Bowel disease, 139

British Rheumatism and Arthritis Association, 174, 175, 203
Brucella, 53
Brucella agglutinins, 187
Brucellosis, 48, 187
Bursae, 83
Bursitis, 85, 91

Caisson disease, 18
Calcification, 91, 93, 101, 138
Calcium, 80, 187
Calcium deficiency, 20
Callosities, 27
Callous formation, 131
Capsule, 7, 9
Carpal tunnel syndrome, 86-87, 200, 224
Carpo-metacarpal joint, 6, 45
Cartilage, 2, 3, 7, 8, 11, 24, 36, 37, 42
Cellulitis, 122
Cervical collar, 78-79
Cervical lordosis, 67
Cervical spine changes, 16
Cervical spondylosis, 73
Cervical traction, 78
Chairs, 158-59, 165
Charcot joints, 51
Charnley arthroplasty, 64
Chiropody, 20, 173
Chloroquine, 217
Chorea, 110, 111
Climatic conditions, 181
Clothing, 174
Clutton's joints, 50
Codeine, 205, 207
Colchicine, 125
Cold therapy, 150
Collagen, 9, 68
Collagen diseases, 10, 96
Condylar joint, 5
Conjunctivitis, 48
Connective tissue, 9
Connective tissue diseases, 10, 96-106
Cord claudication, 72
Corsets, 78
Corticosteroids, 44, 55, 80, 83, 85, 99, 105, 106, 113, 138, 141, 200, 214-16, 233

Costochondral junction, 1
Costo-vertebral joints, 58, 59
Coxsackie virus, 48, 87
Crohn's disease, 14, 139, 192
Cruciate ligaments, 8
Crutches, 161, 174
Crystals, 190
Cysts, 225

Debridement, 224, 227
Decompression operations, 224
Deformity, 177
  flexion, 169-71, 181, 234
  prevention of, 178, 197
Degenerative disease of the spine, 65-81
  anatomy, 65-88
  clinical features, 71-74
  investigations, 74-77
  management, 78
  pathology, 69
  surgery, 81
  treatment, 77-81
Depression, 95, 169, 201, 218
De Quervain's tenosynovitis, 83
Dermatomyositis, 87, 103-5
  clinical features, 104
  definition, 104
  laboratory tests, 104
  treatment, 105
'Devil's grip', 48
Dextropropoxyphene, 206
Diapulse therapy, 150
Diazepam, 80, 171, 218
Diet, 177, 181, 196, 202
Differential agglutination test (DAT), 187
Differential cell count, 189
Dihydrocodeine, 207
Diphtheroids, 22
Disability, 174, 230
Disabled person, 19
Disablement Resettlement Officer, 175
Disc degeneration, 69
Disc prolapse, 71, 72, 77, 80, 81
Discography, 76

Distal interphalangeal joint, 26, 39
District nurse, 201
Dressing aids, 158, 164
Driving postures, 80
'Dropped fingers', 28
Drug induced SLE, 100
Drug therapy, 79-81, 177, 199, 204-22 new forms of, 219
Drugs
  analgesic, 44, 205-8, 220
  analgesic/anti-inflammatory, 44, 208-13, 221
  anti-inflammatory, 44, 213-17
  antimalarial, 99, 138, 217
  cytotoxic, 55, 105
  glossary of, 220
  immunosuppressive, 220
  muscle relaxants, 218
  psychiatric, 218
  toxic effects, 33
  uricosuric, 123, 124
  see also under individual drugs
Dupuytren's contracture, 8, 83
Dysentery, 14, 49

Eburnation, 37
-ectomy, definition, 224
Education of the patient, 173-74
Effusions, 190
Elastin, 9
Elbow joint mobilisation, 156
Electrical therapy, 151
Electrodiagnostic tests, 191-92
Electromyography, 191
Ellipsoid joint, 5
Emotional factors, 22, 110, 181
Employment, 161, 175, 181-82
Enteric infections, 48
Enteropathic arthritis, 139
Epicondylitis, 85
Epidemic myalgia, 87
Epilepsy, 152
Episcleritis, 28
Erythrocyte Sedimentation Rate (ESR), 104, 111, 184
Excision arthroplasty, 227
Exercises, 145-48, 152, 155
  basic forms, 145-46
  purpose, 147
  special type, 147-48
Eyes in rheumatoid arthritis, 28

Faradism, 151
Felty's syndrome, 185
Fenamates, 212
Fenoprofen, 213
Fibrillation, 36
Fibrositis nodules, 87
Fingers
  dropped, 28
  flexion of, 83
  joint mobilisation, 156
  osteoarthrosis, 40
  rheumatoid arthritis, 28
  sausage, 138
  trigger, 28, 83
Flat feet, 131
Flexion deformity, 169-71, 181, 234
Flufenamic acid, 212
Foot disorders, 126-34
  arches, 131
  forefoot, 129
  heel, 134
  hindfoot, 132
  in general disease, 127-29
  local, 129-34
Foot examination, 127
Footwear, 127, 130-32, 171
Fowler's arthroplasty, 227
Frederick the Great of Prussia, 12
Frozen shoulder, 92-93
Fusarium, 13

Garrod's pad, 39
German measles, 47
Giant cell arteritis, 143
Gibbus deformity, 54
Gleno-humeral joint, 89, 93
Glycosuria, 199
Gold, 138, 188, 199-201, 216
Golfer's elbow, 85
Gonococcal complement fixation test (GCFT), 188
Gonorrhoea, 50, 188

Gout, 13, 14, 19, 112, 115-25, 129, 174, 177, 186, 190
  aetiology, 115
  clinical course, 121
  clinical features, 117-21
  diagnosis, 192
  differential diagnosis, 122
  in history, 115
  investigations, 121
  joints involved, 118
  treatment, 122-25

Haematinics, 218
Haematoma formation, 233
Haemoglobin level (Hb), 184
Hallux rigidus, 130
Hallux valgus, 130
Hammer toe, 130, 132
Hand, rheumatoid, 25
Handicap, 19, 167
Harvey, Sir William, 12
Health visitor, 33, 170, 202-3
Heat therapy, 149
Heberden's nodes, 39
Hemiarthroplasty, 229
Hemi-lumbarisation, 66
Hemi-sacralisation, 66
Heredity, 13, 23
Hinge arthroplasties, 230
Hinge joint, 5
Hip joint, 3, 4, 27
  McKee-Farrar arthroplasty, 229
  McMurray osteotomy, 228
  mobilisation, 157
  osteoarthrosis, 27, 41, 45, 177
  replacements, 45
  tuberculous infection, 53
HLA-B27, 61
Home, disability in the, 19
Home conditions, 163, 232
Home modification, 157
Housemaid's knee, 85
Housing, 202
Hubbard tank, 148
Humero-ulnar joint, 5
Hyaluronic acid, 7, 10, 11
Hydrallazine, 100
Hydrocortisone, 83, 91, 93

Hydrotherapy, 64, 148, 170
Hydroxychloroquine, 217
Hyperaemia, 24
Hypertrophic pulmonary osteoarthropathy, 139-41

Ibuprofen, 213
Immune system, 23
Immunosuppressive drugs, 220
Impairment, 167
Indomethacin, 122, 212
Industrial Rehabilitation Unit, 175
Industry, days lost to, 17
Infection, 47, 52
  control of, 176
Infective arthritis, 47-55
Inflammatory effusions, 190
Injections, 200, 201, 216, 218
Injuries, 178
Insomnia, 95, 169
Inter-metacarpal joint, 4
Intervertebral disc, 68, 76
Intra-articular structures, 8
Intra-articular therapy, 55
Ion transfer, 151
Iritis, 58, 61
Iron, 200, 218

Jaccoud's arthropathy, 114
Jaw, receding, 30
Joints
  classification, 1
  loads on, 10
  mobilisation, 156
  structure and function of, 1-11
  surgery, 226
  protection, 155
  synovial (diarthrodial), 2, 3
  types of, 3

Kashin-Beck disease, 12
Keratoderma blenorrhagica, 49
Ketoprofen, 213
Kidneys, 98, 105
Kitchen aids, 164, 174, 175
Knee jerk, 111
Knee joint, 5, 7, 18
  arthroplasty, 230

Knee joint (contd)
  mobilisation, 157
  osteoarthrosis, 38, 41, 227
  osteotomy, 45
  rheumatoid arthritis, 27
Knock-knee, 46, 234

Laboratory investigation, 183-93
LE cells, 185
Leucocytosis, 93
Leucopeania, 185
Leukaemia, 55, 64
Libman-Sacks vegetations, 99
Lifting, 178
Ligaments, 3, 7, 8
Loads on joints, 10
Loom, 162
Lubrication, 7, 10
Lumbar disc, 16, 174
Lumbar lordosis, 59, 67
Lumbar traction, 77
Lumbarisation, 66
Lymph gland biopsy, 191
Lymph nodes, 99

McKee-Farrar arthroplasty, 229
Mackintosh arthroplasty, 229
McMurray osteotomy, 228
Mahler, 12
Massage, 150
Mechanical factors, 177, 181
Median nerve, 224, 232
Mefanamic acid, 212
Meningococci, 54
Menisci, 8
Menopause, 39
Metacarpo-phalangeal joint, 5, 8, 25, 39, 155, 227
Metatarsalgia, 131
Metatarso-phalangeal joint, 27, 118, 127, 129-31, 232
Methocarbamol, 80, 218
Methylprednisolone, 80
Micrognathism, 30
Mobility aids, 174
Mobility assessment, 161
Mobility factor, 232
Morale, 199, 201

Morphine, 208
Mudpacks, 150
Mumps, 47
Muscle, 8
  in rheumatoid arthritis, 28
Muscle biopsy, 191
Muscle pain, 87
Muscle relaxants, 218
Muscle relaxation, 150
Muscle spasm, 87, 110, 218
Muscular rheumatism, 87-88
Myalgia, 47
Mycoplasma, 22
Myelography, 75, 78
Myocarditis, 109

Naproxen, 213
National Health Service expenditure, 19
Nerve conduction studies, 192
Nerve supply, 7
Nodule biopsy, 191
Non-articular rheumatism, 82-88
Non-inflammatory effusions, 190
Non-specific urethritis, 14
Nursing care, 165, 194-203
  community care, 201
  general principles, 194-96
  observation, 197-99
  special procedures, 200-1
  surgery, 234

Occupation, 161, 181-82
Occupational factors, 168
Occupational therapists, 33
Occupational therapy, 153-66, 170
  ankylosing spondylitis, 162
  assessment of patients, 157
  crafts for joint mobilisation, 156-57
  remedial programme, 154
  specific programme, 156
Oesophagus, 102
Oil/wax bath, 149
Opera glass fingers and toes, 138
Opiates, 208
Oral contraceptives, 100
Organisms, 189

Osteoarthrosis, 7, 18, 19, 36-46, 65, 66, 69, 89, 168, 174
  clinical signs, 38
  definition, 36
  diagnosis, 43, 192
  finger, 40
  hand, 25
  hip, 27, 41, 45, 177
  joints involved, 40
  knee, 38, 41, 227
  pathology, 36
  primary, 36, 38
  prognosis, 44
  radiology, 16, 42, 127
  secondary, 36, 41
  surgery, 45
  treatment, 43
  types of, 36
Osteomyelitis, 188
Osteophytes, 37, 74, 75
Osteoporosis, 75, 80
Osteotomy, 224, 227, 233
Overspill pneumonitis, 102
Oxyphenbutazone, 210-12

Pain and pain relief, 80, 196, 205, 230
Pannus, 24
Paracetamol, 205, 206
Patellectomy, 224
Pelvic traction, 77
Pelvis, 1
Penicillamine, 188, 199
D-penicillamine, 219
Penicillin, 17, 100, 107, 112, 176, 177
Pentazocine, 207-8
Periarthritic personality, 96, 169
Periarthritis of the shoulder, 92
Pericarditis, 28
Peripheral neuropathy, 105
Personality factor, 169, 233
Perthes's disease, 41
Pes cavus, 132
Pethidine, 208
Phenacetin, 206
Phenylbutazone, 122, 123, 210-12
Phenytoin, 100
Phosphorus, 187
Physiotherapists, 33

Physiotherapy, 45, 78-79, 144-52, 170, 233
  dangers, 152
  proper use, 144
  types of, 145
Piano-key sign, 27
Pigmentation, 101
Plain joint, 4
Plantar fasciitis, 129, 132
Plastazote, 78
Plaster jackets, 78
Plasters, 171, 196-97
Platelet count, 185
Pobble operation, 129
Podagra, 118
'Poker back', 56, 59
Poliomyelitis, 41
Polyarteritis nodosa, 105-6
  clinical features, 105
  laboratory tests, 106
  treatment, 106
Polymyalgia rheumatica, 141-43
  diagnosis, 143
Polymyositis, 82, 103-5
  clinical features, 104
  definition, 104
  laboratory tests, 104
  treatment, 105
Potter, Dennis, 135-36
Pott's disease, 53
Prednisolone, 105, 106
Pregnancy, 1
Prevention, 176-82
  of deformity, 178, 197
  of symptoms, 181
  public health measures, 176
Probenecid, 123, 177
Procainamide, 100
Propionic acid derivatives, 213
Proteins, 186
Proximal interphalangeal joints, 25, 39
Pseudo-gout, 122
Psoriasis, 14
Psoriatic arthritis, 129, 135-39
  deforming type, 138
  distal type, 136
  identical type, 136

Psoriatic arthritis (*contd*)
  prognosis, 138
  treatment, 138
Psychiatric drugs, 218
Pulley (trochoid) joint, 6
Pus cells, 188, 190
Pyogenic arthritis, 112, 122, 189
Pyrazoles, 210

Radio-active isotopes, 200
Radiology, 192
Radiotherapy, 64
Rancho splint, 225
Raynaud's phenomenon, 98, 101
Reaching aids, 164
Rehabilitation, 153, 154, 167-75, 199, 203, 233
  factors affecting, 167-69
  scope of, 167
Reiter's disease, 48, 49, 132, 177, 187, 188
Remedial programme, 154
Renal calculi, 54
Renal disease, 98, 100
Renal transplantation, 55
Rheumatic diseases, 12-20
  distribution, 12
  prevalence, 12
Rheumatic fever, 13, 17, 88, 107-14, 122, 176-77
  aetiology, 107
  cardiac damage, 109, 112
  cardiac failure, 110, 113
  cardiac manifestations, 114
  clinical features, 109-11
  diagnosis, 111
  diagnostic criteria, 107
  differential diagnosis, 112
  investigations, 111
  laboratory tests, 111
  pathology, 108
  sequelae, 113-14
  treatment, 112
Rheumatic heart disease, 108-9
Rheumatism, non-articular, 82-88
Rheumatoid arthritis, 10, 12, 16, 19, 21-35, 82, 86, 168, 182, 187-90
  aetiology, 22

age factor, 15
anxiety, 169
blood test for, 30
calcium deficiency, 20
clinical findings, 24
complications, 233
course of the disease, 24
definition, 21
diagnosis, 22, 31, 192
education of the patient, 173-74
extra-articular manifestations, 28
eyes, 28
finger, 8, 28, 83
foot, 127
hand, 25
joint infections, 55
juvenile, 29
knee, 27
muscles, 28
osteotomy, 227
pathology, 23
prevention of deformity, 178, 197
prognosis, 34
remedial programme, 155
septic arthritis, 54
toes, 27
treatment, 33, 216, 217, 219, 220
wrist, 27
Rheumatoid disease, 28
Rheumatoid factor, 22, 30, 102, 104, 106, 187, 190
Rheumatoid nodules, 28, 111
Rheumatoid spondylitis, 61
Rotator cuff disease, 91
Rubella, 47

Sacralisation, 66, 69
Sacro-iliac joints, 56, 59, 61
Sacro-iliitis, 135, 138, 139
Saddle (sellar) joint, 6
St Vitus' Dance, 110
Salicylates, 112, 113, 208-10
Salmonella arthritis, 48, 49
Sausage fingers, 138
Scleroderma, 101
Scoliosis, 68
Septic arthritis, 54

Septicaemia, 188
Serum uric acid, See Uric acid
Severely disabled patient, 161
Sexually-transmitted urethritis, 49
Sheep cell agglutination test, 22, 30, 187
Shoes, See Footwear
Short wave diathermy, 150, 152
Shoulder arthroplasty, 230
Shoulder disorders, 89-95
Shoulder girdle, 181
Shoulder-hand syndrome, 94
Shoulder joint, 27, 89
   mobilisation, 156
Shoulder pain, referred, 94-95
Silicone, 45
Skin traction, 77
Slipped disc, 58, 71
Social worker, 33
Spa therapy, 149
Spina bifida, 65
Spina bifida occulta, 65-66
Spinal curvature, 68, 73
Spinal stenosis, 72
Spine, 56
   tuberculous infection, 53
   see also Degenerative disease of the spine
Splenomegaly, 99
Splintage, 165, 171, 196, 197, 225
Spondylolisthesis, 75
Spondylosis, 65
Sportsmen, 41-42, 178
Stand-sit chair, 162
Staphylococci, 55
Sternoclavicular joint, 55
Steroids, 75, 199
Sticks, 161
Still's disease, 29-30, 51, 109
Streptococcal infection, 111, 112, 177
Streptococci, 107, 108
Streptolysin, 111
Streptomycin, 100
Subdeltoid bursitis, 92
Sugar test, 189
Sulphinpyrazone, 123, 177
Sulphonamides, 100, 112, 176, 177
Superior radio-ulnar joint, 6

Surgery, 223-34
   advances in, 223
   complications, 233
   definitions, 224
   factors affecting, 230
   joints, 226
   nursing care, 234
Symphysis pubis, 1
Symptoms, prevention of, 181
Synostosis, 1
Synovectomy, 3, 224, 227, 232
Synovial biopsy, 190
Synovial fluid, 2, 3, 7, 11, 38, 109, 189
Synovial membrane, 3, 9
Synovitis, 23, 37, 47, 48, 51, 56, 58
Synovium, 7, 8, 193
Synthetic lubricants, 45
Syphilis, 50-51, 187
Systemic lupus erythematosus (SLE), 10, 97-103, 185
   aetiology, 97
   blood tests, 99
   cardiovascular involvement, 99
   clinical features, 98-99
   drug induced, 100
   incidence, 97
   laboratory tests, 99
   presentation, 98
   prognosis, 98, 100-1
   renal involvement, 98, 100, 199
   treatment, 99-100
Systemic sclerosis, 101-3
   aetiology, 101
   clinical features, 101
   laboratory tests, 102
   prognosis, 103
   treatment, 103

Telangectasia, 101
Tendon sheaths, 28, 83, 102
Tendons, 8, 9, 91, 102
   surgery, 225
Tennis elbow, 85, 200
Tenosynovitis, 50, 83, 200, 225
Tenotomy, 224
Tetracycline, 100
Thyroid deficiency, 88
Tissue examination, 190-91

243

Tissue procedures, 224
Toes in rheumatoid arthritis, 27
Toilet seat, raised, 158
Tophi, 119, 124, 125
Traction, 77, 78, 151
Transport aids, 162
Trauma, 82
Treadle machines, 163
'Trigger finger', 28, 83
Tuberculosis, 53, 189

Ulcerative colitis, 14, 139
Ulnar deviation, 26
Ulnar styloid, 27
Ultrasonic therapy, 150
Undulant fever, 48
Urate deposits, 120
Urethritis, 48
Uric acid, 115-19, 121-25, 177, 186, 190
Uricosuric drugs, 123, 124
Urine tests, 188, 199-201, 217

Vainio arthroplasty, 227

Varicose veins, 38
Vasculitis, 28
Vasi nervori, 105
Venereal diseases, 177
Ventform traction, 78
Vertebrae, 65, 68
Vertebral column, 65-68
Vichy baths, 148, 150
Vocational training, 175

Walking, 199-200
Washing, 164
Wasserman reaction (WR), 187
Weather factors, 181
Weaving, 162
Wheelchairs, 161, 166
Whipple's disease, 52, 139
White blood count (W.b.c.), 185
Widow's hump, 75
Wrist
  joint mobilisation, 156
  rheumatoid arthritis, 27

X-ray, 16, 42, 61, 192